An Atlas of
ENDOMETRIOSIS

THE ENCYCLOPEDIA OF VISUAL MEDICINE SERIES

An Atlas of
ENDOMETRIOSIS

R. W. Shaw

University of Wales College of Medicine
Cardiff

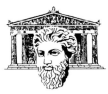

The Parthenon Publishing Group
International Publishers in Medicine, Science & Technology

Casterton Hall, Carnforth,
Lancs, LA6 2LA, UK

One Blue Hill Plaza, Pearl River,
New York 10965, USA

British Library Cataloguing-in-Publication Data
Shaw, Robert W.
  Atlas of Endometriosis. – (Encyclopedia of Visual
  Medicine Series)
  I. Title II. Series
  618.14
  ISBN 1-85070-390-6

Library of Congress Cataloging-in-Publication Data
Shaw, Robert W. (Robert Wayne)
  An atlas of endometriosis/ R. W. Shaw
      p.   cm. – (The Encyclopedia of visual medicine series)
  Includes bibliographical references and index.
  ISBN 1-85070-390-6 : $70.00
  I. Endometriosis–Atlases.   I. Title.   II. Series.
  [DNLM: 1. Endometriosis–atlases. WP 17 S535a]

RG 483. E53S5   1993
618.1'42–dc20
DNLM/DLC
for Library of Congress   92-48868
                                                      CIP

Published in the UK and Europe by
The Parthenon Publishing Group Limited
Casterton Hall, Carnforth
Lancs. LA6 2LA

Published in North America by
The Parthenon Publishing Group Inc.
One Blue Hill Plaza,
PO Box 1564, Pearl River,
New York 10965, USA

Copyright © 1993 Parthenon Publishing Group Ltd

First published 1993

Typeset by AMA Graphics Ltd., Preston
Printed and bound in Great Britain by William Clowes Limited,
Beccles and London

Contents

The Encyclopedia of Visual Medicine Series

Titles currently planned in this series include:

Series Foreword

The art of effective diagnosis is one that relies to a considerable degree – although certainly not exclusively – on the recognition of visual signs and manifestations of disease. The objective of the Series is to provide a practical aid to diagnosis by illustrating and explaining the wide range of visual signs that a physician needs to be aware of in current medical practice.

Whilst the visual manifestations of disease themselves remain constant, the development of new techniques of invasive and non-invasive diagnosis mean that new images are frequently being added to the range of visual material that the diagnostician must be familiar with: ultrasound, radiology, magnetic resonance imaging, endoscopy and photomicrography all provide examples of this kind of material. It is the intention of this Series to document, where appropriate, the result of such techniques and to explain and elucidate their relevance – in addition to documenting all the more standard visual images.

The Series is also distinctive in that individual volumes will focus on carefully selected, specific topics, which can be covered in some detail – rather than on generalized and broadly-based subject areas that could not easily be covered so thoroughly.

The authors contributing to the Series have all been selected for their special expertise in their own chosen fields, their access to outstanding visual material and their ability to explain the significance of it in an effective and lucid way. Finally, particular emphasis is being placed on achieving a very high quality of colour reproduction in the printing process itself in order to do full justice to the wide variety of visual images presented.

It is hoped that this carefully structured and systematic approach to the visually significant aspects of medicine will make a valuable and ongoing contribution to good diagnostic practice.

Preface

Endometriosis presents a unique clinical and scientific challenge for both gynaecologists and basic clinical scientists. It remains one of the most frequently encountered pathologies diagnosed amongst gynaecological patients. It would seem that it has been diagnosed with increased frequency in the last decade, and yet, for many patients, we are unsure of the significance of its presence in relationship to its contribution towards that individual's symptomatology.

Conclusive recognition of endometriosis is necessary for appropriate diagnosis, to enable informed consent and planning of relevant and appropriate therapy for that individual patient. Whilst the classical powder-burn puckered bluish/black lesions are recognized as the hallmark of the presence of endometriosis, in recent years more subtle appearances have been documented and recognized. These would seem to be more common and possibly even more active than the typical black lesions.

This volume contains a series of photographs illustrating the visual appearance of endometriosis, as well as a collection of histopathological pictures from documented cases of endometriosis involving the peritoneum, the ovary, other commonly involved pelvic organs and of some less common extrapelvic and extragenital sites.

In the collection of this series of photographs and histopathological pictures, I am indebted to several colleagues and friends in addition to my patients. Dr Peter Lindsay MRCOG, who was my Endometriosis Clinical Research Fellow (1990–92) collected many of the laparoscopic photographs.

Dr Julie Crow (Senior Lecturer, Department of Histopathology, Royal Free Hospital, School of Medicine) prepared the histopathological slides from the many biopsies and specimens we sent her from patients under my care. In addition, Mr Chris Sutton (Consultant Gynaecologist, Guildford), Mr David Bromham (Senior Lecturer, St. James Hospital, Leeds) and Professor Jacques Donnez (St. Luc Hospital, Brussels) allowed me to utilize some of their slides which are appropriately acknowledged in the text.

The text of this Atlas is not meant to represent a definitive review of endometriosis in itself. This would require a large textbook to give full justification to our current understanding of the aetiology and pathogenesis, the association of the disease with symptomatology, and a full appropriate review of the treatment options. The text is merely meant to present a current synopsis and to refer the reader on to more definitive reviews. I hope that the Atlas will provide the gynaecologist with an interesting text to read and a large (although by no means entirely fully comprehensive) collection of visual appearances of endometriosis, which may help the laparoscopist to identify lesions he or she may encounter in their own patients and serve as a useful teaching aid for gynaecologists in training.

Section 1 A Review of Endometriosis

General introduction

Endometriosis is one of the commonest benign gynaecological conditions. It has been estimated to be present in between 10 and 25% of women presenting with gynaecological symptoms in the United Kingdom and the USA. This incidence is based on finding its presence in patients who have undergone laparoscopy for diagnostic indications[1,2]. Although it is an extremely common condition, there is much that is still not understood and the condition still arouses much interest and controversy.

The definition of endometriosis may seem to be deceptively simple: 'the presence of functional endometrial tissue outside the uterine cavity'. Clinical diagnosis is made usually by laparoscopic observations of small or large haemorrhagic or fibrotic foci on the pelvic peritoneum or serosal surface of the pelvic organs. This ectopic endometrial tissue responds to ovarian hormones undergoing cyclical changes which, whilst not exactly comparable to those seen in the eutopic endometrium, are closely similar. The cyclical bleeding from the endometriotic deposit appears to contribute to the induction of a local inflammatory reaction, fibrous adhesion formation, and, in the case of deep ovarian implants, leads to the formation of endometriomas or 'chocolate cysts'.

From the turn of the century, there has been substantial interest in this fascinating disease but still relatively little scientific data concerning its cause, natural history and its relationship to subfertility. Endometriosis commonly affects women during their childbearing years. In the main, this reflects deleterious social, sexual and reproductive consequences. The disease represents a major clinical problem from both a diagnostic viewpoint and as a consumer of a significant proportion of health care expenditures in gynaecological care. It is not known why some women acquire this disease, but it has been well established that its persistence and spread are dependent upon the cyclical secretion of steroid hormones from the ovaries.

Epidemiology

Endometriosis is found almost exclusively in women in the reproductive age group. It can be diagnosed conclusively only by surgical intervention and, as some women are asymptomatic, we can only guess at its true rate of occurrence in the population. The incidence of endometriosis is, therefore, unknown but prevalence data in specific groups are quoted frequently. These are shown in Table 1. From this information, we can estimate the prevalence of endometriosis amongst women of reproductive age as being at least 1%. It has been suggested that the frequency of this disease has increased in recent years. However, one view is that this merely reflects the greater use of diagnostic laparoscopy and an increasing recognition of the more subtle appearances of endometriosis as viewed laparoscopically, many features of which would have been ignored a decade ago. Although endometriosis is primarily a disease of the reproductive years, it has been described both in adolescent and postmenopausal women, and there seems to be no association between age and severity of the disease process or symptomatology.

Table I Prevalence of endometriosis in specific gynaecological patient groups

Women undergoing tubal sterilization[3]	2%
Women with affected first-degree relatives[4]	7%
Infertile women[5]	15–25%
Women with surgically removed ovaries[6]	17%
At diagnostic laparoscopy[7]	0–53%
At gynaecological laparotomy[7]	0.1–50%
In unexplained infertility[5]	70–80%

Aetiology: factors involved in pathogenesis

The precise aetiology of endometriosis still remains unknown. It has often been called the disease of theories because of the many postulated theories encompassed to explain its pathogenesis. During the first half of this century, several theories were proposed to explain the process through which endometriosis develops. Subsequently, clinical and experimental evidence has accumulated to support each of these concepts; however, no single theory can explain the location of endometriotic deposits in all of the sites reported.

Menstrual regurgitation and implantation
Sampson in 1927 suggested that endometriosis developed as a result of menstrual regurgitation and subsequent implantation of endometrial tissue on the peritoneal surface[8]. In support of this theory, experimental endometriosis has been induced in animals by placement of menstrual fluid or endometrial tissue in the peritoneal cavity. In addition, endometriosis has been described in young girls in association with abnormalities of the genital tract causing obstruction to the outflow of menstrual fluid[9].

Retrograde menstruation through the Fallopian tubes is, however, a common finding at laparoscopy if performed during the perimenstrual period[10], and, therefore, some other mechanism, which may be immunological, must account for the subsequent development of endometriosis in susceptible individuals.

Genetic and immunological factors
Dmowski and colleagues suggested that genetic and immunological factors may alter the susceptibility of a woman to allow her to develop endometriosis[11]. Indeed, these workers demonstrated a decreased cellular immunity to endometriotic tissue in women with endometriosis. Another group of workers[4] demonstrated an increased incidence of endometriosis in first-degree relatives of patients with the disorder compared to a control group, and racial differences also exist, with a reported increased prevalence amongst Oriental women and a lower prevalence in patients of Negroid origin.

Vascular and lymphatic spread
Vascular and lymphatic embolization to distant sites has been demonstrated and explains the rare finding of endometriosis in sites outside the peritoneal cavity, e.g. joints, skin, lung and kidney.

Transformation of coelomic epithelium
The cells lining the Müllerian duct arise from primitive cells which differentiate into peritoneal cells and the cells on the surface of the ovaries. It is proposed that these adult cells undergo de-differentiation back to their primitive origin and then transform into endometrial cells[12]. This is an attractive theory than can

explain the occurrence of endometriosis in nearly all ectopic sites due to the presence of aberrant Müllerian cells. The transformation into endometrial cells may be due to hormonal stimuli of ovarian origin, other chemical substances liberated from the uterine endometrium (induction concept, see reference 13), or to inflammatory irritation.

Almost certainly, an interaction between one or more of these factors is necessary to allow the initial development and then continued growth of an endometriotic implant (see Figure A).

The probability that an individual woman will develop endometriosis can be viewed in quantitative terms by familial factors, delaying of childbearing and increasing the cumulative menstrual exposure appearing to enhance the development of the disease. The almost universal finding of retrograde menstruation and the inherent ability of pelvic tissue to support endometrial transplantation will allow virtually any woman the opportunity to develop the disease. Factors that determine the degree of retrograde menstruation remain to be elucidated and immunological/genetic factors may affect a patient's susceptibility to allow the implantation of these exfoliated endometrial cells.

Symptoms

Symptoms in patients with endometriosis are extremely variable. The symptoms may vary depending upon the site of the ectopic endometrium, but what is apparent is that the extent of the disease does not necessarily bear any relation to the intensity of the symptoms. Indeed, the disease may be a coincidental finding during surgery or investigation for other gynaecological conditions (most commonly infertility).

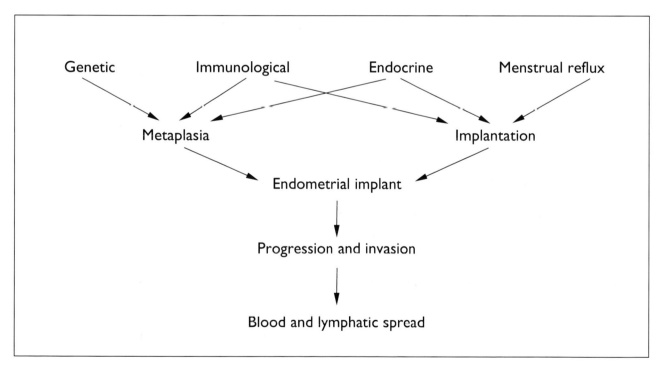

Figure A Suggested aetiological interactions in the formation of an endometriotic implant

Table 2 Symptoms of endometriosis in relationship to site of endometriotic implants

Site	Symptoms
Female reproductive tract	dysmenorrhoea lower abdominal and pelvic pain dyspareunia infertility menstrual irregularity rupture/torsion endometrioma low back pain
Gastrointestinal tract	cyclical tenesmus/rectal bleeding diarrhoea colonic obstruction
Urinary tract	cyclical haematuria/pain ureteral obstruction
Surgical scars, umbilicus	cyclical pain and bleeding
Lung	cyclical haemoptysis

Further research is perhaps necessary to establish whether specific subtle lesions of endometriosis, particularly the haemorrhagic and red papular lesions, are related more specifically to certain symptoms and whether the deep infiltrating lesions with marked surrounding fibrotic reaction are an explanation for persistence of the problem. A variety of symptoms of endometriosis related to the siting of the deposits is summarized in Table 2.

It can be seen from this table that many of these symptoms are shared by a number of common gynaecological disorders or other disorders of the gastrointestinal/urogenital system. Because of this cross-over, many patients with endometriosis have delayed diagnosis of their condition and are often treated for other disorders prior to the definitive diagnosis of endometriosis being made. Perhaps one of the most pertinent diagnostic pointers for the clinician in terms of symptomatology is the onset or increased severity of symptoms in the premenstrual and menstrual phases of the cycle. This association of symptoms, together with occurrence of cyclical haemorrhage and/or tenderness, are often pathognomonic of endometriosis.

Endometriosis and infertility

There exists an association between endometriosis and infertility which occurs in 30–40% of patients suffering with endometriosis[14]. The pathogenesis of infertility in patients with endometriosis is often multifactorial and thus the direct relevance to contribution by the presence of a few small endometriotic deposits may be difficult to determine. It is perhaps more readily explainable in patients with more severe stages of endometriosis in which there is obvious anatomical distortion, for example, periadnexal adhesions or destruction of ovarian tissue by endometrioma. These result in mechanical factors, which may then interfere with the release or pick-up of oocytes. However, when only minimal endometriosis is found in patients complaining of infertility, the cause and effect of the relationship is more difficult to understand. A number of possible mechanisms have been postulated, such as various endocrine disorders (including anovulation), uterine endometrial antibodies, unruptured luteinized follicle syndrome, prostaglandin-induced luteolysis, oocyte maturation defects, prostaglandin-induced alteration of tubal cilial motility, and disorders of coital function. These are summarized in Table 3.

Currently, no simple explanation can be proposed for infertility in the presence of only mild or minimal endometriosis. Many investigators state that it is controversial as to whether such cases benefit from any form of treatment, although most clinicians would offer therapy to patients if there are any other associated symptoms of endometriosis. One argument for offering therapy is perhaps on the grounds that treatment in the early stages of endometriosis may prevent further progress of the disease, which may indeed jeopardize future fertility by the forma-

Table 3 Possible mechanisms of infertility causation with mild/minimal endometriosis

Ovarian function	endocrinopathies anovulation luteinized unruptured follicle syndrome altered prolactin secretion luteolysis caused by prosta- glandin F_2 oocyte maturation defects
Tubal function	prostaglandin-induced alteration of tubal and/or cilial motility
Coital function/ frequency	dyspareunia – reduced frequency/penetration problems
Spermatozoal function	increased phagocytosis by activated macrophages inactivation by antibodies
Implantation	interference from endometrial antibodies luteal phase defects
Early pregnancy loss	prostaglandin-induced immune response increased early spontaneous abortion

tion of adhesions and ovarian/tubal fixity with compromise of function.

A recent extensive review of this topic has been summarized by Thomas[15]. His conclusions were that 'the balance of evidence is that, apart from mechanical damage, endometriosis does not cause infertility'. Current knowledge of the natural history of the disease and the impact of drug therapy upon it, does not allow us to recommend that the finding of mild endometriosis *per se* requires treatment. However, there is evidence that medical or surgical treatment is beneficial if it involves the lysis of peritubal and periovarian adhesions or the removal of ovarian endometriomas.

Frequency of symptoms

Table 4 summarizes the frequency of the commoner symptoms of endometriosis, compiled primarily from our own clinical experience but also from published data in the literature.

Diagnosis

The possibility of endometriosis should be a differential diagnostic consideration in any patient presenting with infertility or with worsening dysmenorrhoea, pelvic pain, dyspareunia or other associated cyclical symptoms, particularly related to the gastrointestinal or urogenital system.

Clinical findings

Pelvic endometriosis   Clinical findings in endometriosis are markedly variable. In mild cases, routine gynaecological examination is likely to reveal no abnormality. A common feature on bimanual pelvic examination is that of discomfort, especially if performed during the premenstrual phase. It may be possible to palpate induration and tenderness in the uterosacral ligaments when these are involved. These features are demonstrated perhaps most clearly by a combined vaginal and rectal examination.

Table 4 Frequency of commoner symptoms of endometriosis, as composed from analysis of 500 of my own patients and published data[16-19]

Symptom	Likely frequency (%)
Dysmenorrhoea	60 – 80
Pelvic pain	30 – 50
Infertility	30 – 40
Dyspareunia	25 – 40
Menstrual irregularities	10 – 20
Cyclical dysuria/haematuria	1 – 2
Dyschesia (cyclic)	1 – 2
Rectal bleeding (cyclic)	< 1

If the posterior cul-de-sac is involved extensively, the uterus will become fixed in retroversion and the adnexae will appear immobile.

Ovarian endometriosis Deep involvement of the ovaries, with formation of cystic endometriomas, may be suspected from unilateral adnexal tenderness, although palpation of a cyst less than 5 cm in diameter may be difficult. The finding of a defined adnexal mass or indeed unilateral adnexal pathology with tenderness in a patient of reproductive age is always suggestive of endometriosis.

Endometriosis involving other organs When the mucosa of the rectum, sigmoid or bladder are involved, there may be overt haemorrhage, or haemorrhagic lesions may be visible if viewed perimenstrually. However, in many instances, even with deep-seated involvement, there is no obvious mucosal lesion. It may be only after bimanual examination that areas of nodularity and fibrosis can be localized within these organs, or endometriosis is suspected from observation of the involvement of the serosal surface of the bladder or bowel with endometriotic implants.

For specific diagnosis in the majority of instances, both visualization and biopsy of the lesions are essential, either at laparoscopy and/or laparotomy.

Serum markers

Attempts have been made to use specific serum markers for endometriosis. The most widely used has been the measurement by a mononuclear antibody to CA125, which was raised against an ovarian epithelial tumour antigen OC125. Serum levels of CA125 have been found to be elevated in 80% of patients with epithelial ovarian cancer but in less than 2% of normal women[20]. Barbieri and colleagues also found that patients with endometriosis tended to have higher serum levels than normal patients[20]. However, further studies have demonstrated that, whilst a significant proportion of patients with Revised American Fertility Society[21] Stages 3 and 4 of the disease have elevated levels, patients with mild and minimal stages of endometriosis have levels within the normal range. Thus, the specificity when using serum CA125 as a screen for the presence of endometriosis is poor. Our own studies found that, whilst measurement of serum CA125 may not be helpful in the initial diagnosis of endometriosis, in patients in whom it was found to be elevated, serial monitoring of levels was a pointer for the recurrence of the disease during follow-up[22].

Classification

Most medical classifications are descriptive, particularly those devised by pathologists and physiologists who are interested in the aetiology and pathophysiology of specific diseases. As clinicians concerned with the management of patients, we have other demands of classification systems. This is certainly true in the case of endometriosis and presents us with significant problems. We need a classification system to be:

> simple,
> rapid,
> objective (correlating with the volume of tissue perhaps),
> reproducible,
> containing some symptom assessment,
> of good prognostic value,
> correlated with lesion changes on treatment.

In this respect, the major problem with endometriosis is that there appears to be no direct correlation between the volume of tissue and the severity of symptoms related to either pain or infertility. The many vastly different appearances of endometriosis will also make achievement of an ideal classification difficult. To date, a number of classification systems have been described. These include those by Acosta and colleagues in 1973[23], Kistner and colleagues in 1977[24], and the American Fertility Classification (AFS) of 1979[25] and its modification in 1985[21]. Primarily, all these classifications divide endometriosis into various

The American Fertility Society Revised Classification of endometriosis

Patient's Name _____ Date _____

Stage I   (Minimal)   1–5   Laparoscopy _____ Laparotomy _____ Photography _____
Stage II   (Mild)   6–15   Recommended Treatment _____
Stage III (Moderate)   16–40   _____
Stage IV   (Severe)   > 40   _____

Total _____   Prognosis _____

	ENDOMETRIOSIS		< 1 cm	1–3 cm	> 3 cm
PERITONEUM		Superficial	1	2	4
		Deep	2	4	6
OVARY	R	Superficial	1	2	4
		Deep	4	16	20
	L	Superficial	1	2	4
		Deep	4	16	20
	POSTERIOR CUL-DE-SAC OBLITERATION		Partial		Complete
			4		40
	ADHESIONS		< 1/3 Enclosure	1/3–2/3 Enclosure	> 2/3 Enclosure
OVARY	R	Filmy	1	2	4
		Dense	4	8	16
	L	Filmy	1	2	4
		Dense	4	8	16
TUBE	R	Filmy	1	2	4
		Dense	4*	8*	16
	L	Filmy	1	2	4
		Dense	4*	8*	16

* If the fimbriated end of the Fallopian tube is completely enclosed, change the point assignment to 16.

Additional Endometriosis: Associated Pathology: _____
_____   _____
_____   _____
_____   _____

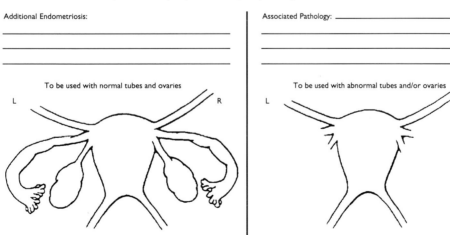

To be used with normal tubes and ovaries   To be used with abnormal tubes and/or ovaries

Figure B   The American Fertility Society Revised Classification of endometriosis[21]

stages with the stage of severity increasing with involvement of the ovaries and with adhesion formation. All systems were basically aimed at trying to correlate increasing severity of the disease with subsequent fertility outcome. However, for many patients, the recurrent, long-standing nature of the disease is one of pain. This factor needs to be incorporated to try to achieve a classification scheme which may be predictive for pain and/or recurrence, rather than trying merely to predict fertility. A single classification incorporating all of these goals may be impossible. To date, the Revised AFS is used most commonly in investigative studies and at least allows a comparison between the results published by different authors. This is illustrated in Figure B.

In addition to the Revised AFS system, it may be helpful to chart carefully the exact sites of all lesions and their sizes, as used in the scheme of additive diameters of implants, described by Doberl and colleagues[26]. This may give a simple quantitative valuation of alteration in the 'volume' of the disease process, although not the activity of lesion/implants, following surgical or medical intervention. One major shortcoming of the Revised AFS recording system is the high scores which are achieved in the presence of adhesions. This means that the patient remains in a moderate or severe stage of the disease, even though the active disease process has been eliminated and only the adhesions persist. This may be relevant to infertility, but is less helpful in the management of chronic pain.

Currently, then, endometriosis is diagnosed from both its typical and atypical laparoscopic appearances and histological features. Both of these will be discussed in the next section.

Laparoscopic appearances

The diagnosis of endometriosis is often made by the observation of the classical powder burn, puckered black or bluish lesion. This is certainly the easiest to see and document. However, during recent years, the different laparoscopic appearances of peritoneal endometriosis have been studied and correlated with morphological characteristics. In addition to the typical lesions, laparoscopic appearances include:

> areas of hypervascularization,
> yellow/brown pigmentation,
> petechial blood-like red lesions,
> clear lesions (often extremely small),
> pseudoperitoneal pockets,
> adhesions, particularly in the ovarian fossa and on the posterior aspect of the ovary.

Careful and serial histological examination of these varying types of lesions has identified endometriotic elements within all such lesions in varying percentages of cases[27–29]

Types of lesions

Classical implants
The classical implant is a nodular lesion characterized by a varying degree of fibrosis and pigmentation, such that the colour may vary from white to brown or black. Histological examination of biopsies from such lesions shows glandular tissue in approximately 50%.

The endometrial tissue is represented by glandular epithelium surrounded by stroma. The glandular epithelium shows varying degrees of activity, but is frequently inactive with no apparent changes throughout the menstrual cycle.

Vesicular implants
The vesicular implants are small lesions whose diameter is less than 5 mm and may occur singly or as multiple lesions in clusters. These implants are characterized by a prominent vascularization and are frequently red in appearance because of a haemorrhagic admixture. There may also be increased vascularization in the surrounding peritoneal tissue. The endometrial tissue shows the presence of surface epithelium covering a highly vascularized stroma. Fluid accumulates between the surface of the implant and the overlying peritoneum, resulting in blister or vesicle/bleb formation.

White vesicular lesions may also be seen when there is an absence of bleeding, and the vast majority have histological proof of the presence of endometriotic tissue. These may well represent very early stages in the development of a lesion before vascularization has been established fully and haemorrhage ensues.

Papular implants

The papular implant is another small lesion with a diameter of less than 5 mm and again occurs singly or in clusters. The colour of these lesions is usually whitish or occasionally yellow. Histologically, cystic glandular structures with stroma are found enclosed in the subperitoneal tissue. Often vascularization of the peritoneum can be seen overlying the implant, and an accumulation of secretory products results in a cystic structure to the implant, the cyst fluid having a whitish or yellow opaque colour.

Haemorrhagic lesions

The haemorrhagic lesions develop when implants have a surface epithelium covered by stroma with a good vascular supply. Proliferation, secretion and vesicle formation occur with these lesions, and they haemorrhage perimenstrually. Haemorrhagic lesions represent perhaps one of the more active types of lesions.

Nodular lesions

Papular, nodular lesions have no surface epithelium and their components show proliferation and vasodilatation only during the menstrual cycle and usually do not reach full secretory activity. There is no menstrual bleeding within the implants.

Healed implants

Healed implants may still contain cystic glands but these are scant and there is no stroma. The healed implants are surrounded by connective tissue and present as nodular or fibrotic, scarified areas.

Evolution of lesions

Many of the detailed studies and much of the evaluation of the differing types of implant have been performed by Brosens and co-workers (for review, see reference 30).

Colour and direct appearance are the important macroscopic features of endometriosis. Data have been published suggesting a correlation between the patients' age and colour and type of implants visualized[29]. This study showed younger women (less than 25 years of age) to have a preponderance of non-pigmented lesions, whilst older women (over 30 years of age) tended to have more pigmented lesions, as well as more advanced disease.

It is not uncommon to see a multitude of different types of lesions within the same patient and the varying appearances described may well represent change in the evolution of the deposit. Enclosed active lesions may heal, depending on regression of the stromal component and the increasing connective tissue fibrosis. Flattening and evolutionary changes in the glandular epithelium are characteristic of a healed lesion. Frequently, glandular tissue is not found in white fibrotic 'healed lesions'.

The haemorrhagic vesicle is likely to develop into a white or opaque papular implant. Epithelial tufts in the active gland can form polypoidal structures emerging on the surface of the implant, producing the haemorrhagic vesicle. Vascularized polyps respond like superficial endometrium to ovarian hormones, resulting in vascular necrosis at the time of menstruation. These changes induce inflammatory reaction and fibroreactive tissue in the surrounding tissues. Hence, these modify the free haemorrhagic implant, inducing a surface covering to the active implant. The implant may then either continue to grow and become a deep implant, leading possibly to infiltration, or conversely it may undergo spontaneous healing if hormonal and vascular support are reduced and fibrosis predominates.

Infiltrating lesions

Infiltrating, deep lesions may be easier to palpate than to see laparoscopically.

It has been found difficult to develop visual criteria for distinguishing deep infiltration from superficial disease by surface observation seen at laparoscopy. Infiltrating endometriosis (adenomyoma) and the difficulties it presents were noted by Sampson in 1921[31]. In these deep lesions, there is a combination of varying amounts of fibromuscular scar and the glands and stroma of endometriosis. The degree of penetration can vary from as little as 2–3 mm in the majority of lesions to more than 5 mm as found in 25% of lesions.

Deep disease is generally suspected when there are palpable nodules associated with focal tenderness on clinical examination. The presence of the disease can be more readily confirmed by examination under anaesthesia for these palpable nodules. This is best performed by careful palpation of the cul-de-sac, uterosacral ligaments and rectovaginal septum.

Importance of adequate laparoscopic examination

It is apparent that endometriosis has a wide variety of visual appearances and only careful laparoscopic assessment of the pelvis will reveal these features.

In the majority of instances, the laparoscopic appearances of endometriotic lesions are quite characteristic and diagnosis in most cases is simple, without the need for a biopsy. It is more difficult with the non-pigmented and opacified lesions, in which a biopsy may well be necessary to confirm diagnosis. The clinician should look for bluish black implants or papules varying in colour, on or under the peritoneal surface and for deep infiltrating lesions in the cul-de-sac, on and around the uterosacral ligaments and the posterior wall of the uterus and rectovaginal septum.

The most frequent sites of endometriotic involvement within the pelvis are summarized in Table 5.

Table 5 Frequency of location of endometriotic implants in the pelvis (from review of 500 consecutive cases, many individuals having multiple sites of involvement)

Site	Percentages
Uterosacral ligaments	63
Ovaries	
superficial	56
deep (endometrioma)	19.5
Ovarian fossae	32.5
Anterior vesicle pouch	21.5
Pouch of Douglas	18.5
Broad ligament	7.5
Intestines	5.0
Fallopian tube	
mesosalpinx	4.5
salpingitis ischmica nodosa	3.0
Uterus	4.5

Minimal endometriosis can be difficult to diagnose, and in many instances it will be necessary to aspirate the pouch of Douglas of any fluid to be certain that any lesions are not missed. In addition, it is imperative to examine the anterior cul-de-sac over the bladder and peritoneum covering the ovarian fossa.

With advanced endometriosis and massive adhesion formation between the reproductive and neighbouring organs, it may become difficult or impossible to identify the lesions of endometriosis. Usually, however, in such cases, typical lesions of the disease are visible in some area within the pelvis to enable confirmation of the disease.

Histological features

Endometriosis is histologically defined by the presence of endometrial glands and stroma in regions outwith the uterine cavity. There appear to be a number of different histological types of implants, which may well represent different stages in the evolution of the disease and may even be associated with differing pathophysiology and symptoms. Ever since Sampson published his series of articles between 1921 and 1940[8, 31–33], we know that endometriosis may present with diverse clinical and histological features. Sampson described chocolate cysts, blebs, adenomyomatous infiltration of the rectovaginal septum, adhesions (particularly those on the posterior surface of the ovaries), red raspberry, purple-raspberry or bluish lesions on the peritoneum, peritoneal pockets and cancerous changes arising in endometriotic deposits. What, then, are the histological characteristics associated with the laparoscopic appearances of these varying lesions?

Microanatomical subtypes

Three microanatomical types of peritoneal endometriosis have been described[34], using a combination of histology and scanning electronmicroscopy.

Submesothelial

This is characterized by multiple or single endometriotic polyps measuring between 200 and 700 μm in diameter. The polyps are sited under a mesothelial vesicle, the polyp surface being covered by rounded cuboidal non-ciliated cells bearing microvilli and a few isolated ciliated cells. Glandular openings are not seen. Histological sectioning of the polyp reveals the presence of highly vascularized stroma beneath the surface epithelium. The stromal tissue may extend further to the neighbouring peritoneal tissue, and serial sectioning will indicate that the polyps are in continuity with glands at the base of the polyp. Hence, the surface epithelium of the polyp is, as occurs in the surface epithelium of the endometrium, an extension of the glandular epithelium.

Intraepithelial

In this type, the endometrial surface epithelium replaces the mesothelium. Ciliated cells can be identified by scanning electronmicroscopy and, at the transition of the surrounding mesothelium, these epithelial cells then become flattened. In this instance, the lesion is a true intraperitoneal implant and glandular structures may be present or absent.

Subperitoneal

The third type of implant is not detectable by scanning electronmicroscopy as it is enclosed in the subperitoneal tissue. Lesions are shown to include glands and stroma but no surface epithelium. The subperitoneal subgroup represents the classical definition of endometriosis.

These three microanatomical types of endometriotic implants are characterized on the basis of their relationship with the peritoneum and their endometrial glandular components. Commonly, these small lesions do not have well defined stroma, and perhaps represent the early stages of the development of lesions prior to the induction of differentiation of tissues to form stroma, collection within the gland of components of fresh and old haemorrhage, infiltration of macrophages often laden with haemosiderin and the presence of fibrosis, scarring and localized healing within the periphery of lesions – all features usually deemed essential in the histological diagnosis of endometriosis.

The importance of stroma in endometriotic tissue is of vital importance to the survival of the endometriotic glands. During healing, when the fibrotic tissue grows into the endometriotic lesions, it will irradicate the stroma but will never grow into the epithelial structures. In addition, when the stroma has disappeared, the epithelial structures are actually formed and changed to atypical cellular patterns; they appear to be no longer responsive to the cyclical ovarian hormonal changes.

Cyclical changes and steroid receptors

Cyclical histological changes in ectopic implants have been reported[35]. The implants appear to go through cyclical changes similar but not identical to those of the eutopic uterine glands. From both histological and electronmicroscopic studies, these functional changes in the endometriotic glands do not proceed as clearly or as uniformly as in the uterine mucosa[36].

Oestrogen receptors, progesterone receptors and androgen receptors are measurable in endometriotic tissue. Oestrogen receptors are at a lower level than in the endometrium and androgen receptors in the

same range as in the endometrium. In endometriotic deposits, the oestrogen receptor levels appear not to change during the menstrual cycle in such a pronounced manner as in the endometrium. Whilst the endometrial oestrogen receptors are biologically active, the response to hormonal influence is different compared to that in the endometrium, indicating a different regulating mechanism of the steroid receptor function. Studies on progesterone receptors vary, depending on the binding techniques or immunoassays utilized, but indicate a high level of biologically inactive progesterone receptors in endometriotic tissue. These changes again provide additional evidence that the hormonal control of endometriotic tissue is different from that in uterine endometrium, and may explain why a hormonal approach to treatment may not induce comparable changes in all implants (for a review see references 37 and 38).

Conventional histological subtypes

Histological studies of the overt peritoneal lesions of endometriosis lead to subdivision into three main types.

Free implants

These have a polyp or cauliflower structure and grow along the surface or cover a cystic structure characterized by the presence of a surface epithelium supported by endometrial stroma. Endometrial glands may be present or absent. Cyclical changes with both secretory change and menstrual bleeding have been noted in these free implants, making them sensitive to hormonal suppressive therapy.

Enclosed implants

These implants have no surface epithelium and are located within tissue, or are part of the free-growing lesion. They may present as wedge-shaped extensions of stroma (ramification), often deep in local tissue, connecting lesions with each other. During the

Table 6 Histological characteristics of endometriotic implants and their laparoscopic appearance (modified from reference 30)

Histological type	Laparoscopic appearance	Components	Hormonal response
Free	haemorrhagic vesicle/bleb	surface epithelium, glands and stroma	proliferative, secretory and menstrual changes
Enclosed	papule and (later) nodules	glands and stroma	proliferative, variable secretory, no menstruation
Healed	white nodule or flattened fibrotic scar	glands only	no response

menstrual cycle, changes occur only in the minority of cases, and late secretory change or menstrual bleeding is not seen. Both capillary and venous dilatation are seen during the luteal phase, but no necrosis or bleeding occurs at the time of menstruation. Thus, they act rather like basal endometrium and are likely to be only partially responsive to a hormonal treatment approach.

Healed lesions
These are characterized by cystically dilated glands containing a thin glandular epithelium, supported by small numbers of fusiform, stromal cells and surrounded by connective tissue. The absence of functional stromal tissue, and the enclosure of the implants by scar tissue, make the lesions insensitive to hormonal stimuli.

The histological characteristics of the varying endometriotic implants and associated laparoscopic appearances are summarized in Table 6.

Ovarian endometriosis

When involvement of the ovary occurs, endometriosis presents either as a superficial form, as haemorrhagic lesions or, in a more severe form, as a haemorrhagic cyst. Both types of ovarian endometriosis are associated commonly with adhesion formation.

Superficial endometriosis

Superficial lesions can occur on all sides of the ovary and have the varying appearances as seen with involvement of the peritoneum. Common superficial haemorrhagic lesions are red vesicles or blebs, and the blue-black characteristic lesions. Less commonly, only yellowish-brown lesions are seen. Occasionally, there are clear papules, but it is essential that there should be other features of endometriosis present in the ovary before endometriosis is diagnosed, since these clear papules can be confused very commonly with Walthard's rests. It would, therefore, be advisable, in the absence of the other features of endometriosis, to take biopsies of such lesions and not make the diagnosis of endometriosis merely on the visual features alone. It is particularly important to examine all aspects of the ovary, particularly the posterior surface, so as not to miss the features of endometriosis.

Haemorrhagic lesions are commonly associated with adhesion formation, sometimes covering a significant proportion of the ovary. The adhesions can be hard to detect by laparoscopy if they are avascular, transparent or in their early stages of development. This is particularly so when they are on the posterior aspect of the ovary. The histopathological features of superficial ovarian endometriosis are as for those of peritoneal endometriosis previously described.

Deep endometriosis of the ovary: endometrioma

The word 'endometrioma' is used to describe an endometriotic cyst of the ovary. Another term in widespread use is 'chocolate cyst', because of the characteristic dark brown or chocolate-coloured content of the cyst. However, this term can be misleading; since many haemorrhagic cysts are functional cysts – corpora lutea in particular – it is as well to look for the presence of other signs of pelvic endometriosis. In addition, aspiration of the chocolate content of the cyst can aid diagnosis. Other features, such as the site of the cyst on the lateral surface of the ovary, haemorrhagic adhesions and the puckering scar formation, are other indicative features of an endometriotic cyst. Commonly, haemorrhagic cysts of other origin contain large blood clots or even fresh haemorrhage which is unlikely to be present with endometriosis. However, frequently at laparoscopy these characteristics can be lacking, making it impossible to diagnose the origin of the cyst exactly as endometriosis without histological proof.

To aid diagnosis at laparoscopy, the cyst should be aspirated and the cyst cavity irrigated for direct observation of the wall. This commonly shows a uniform white fibrotic appearance but with hypervascularized, haemorrhagic foci in the more active cysts. The haemorrhagic content of the cyst is likely to originate from chronic bleeding from these small areas of free endometriosis.

Histological features of ovarian endometriomas

The histology of an endometrioma is characterized by a wide variation in the endometriotic tissue present. The cyst wall can be lined by free endometrial tissue histologically and functionally similar to that of eutopic endometrium. In many instances, however, particularly with long-standing presence of endometriomas, all traces of endometrial tissue may be lost and the wall of the cyst becomes covered by thickened fibrotic reactive tissue. In between 25 and 35% of cases, no specific histopathological features typical of endometriotic glandular components can be found.

Formation of endometriomas

In the genesis of an endometrioma, it would seem that the lesion commences on the outer surface of the ovary. As it grows larger, the ovarian cortex becomes inverted such that, in most endometriomas, the outside of the chocolate cyst is attached to the outside of the ovary which has become internalized. Frequent leakage from the cyst wall leads commonly to adhesion formation around endometriomas, particularly on the posterior surface of the ovary and in the ovarian fossa or to the posterior aspect of the broad ligament. The inverted ovarian cortex frequently becomes adherent to the parametrium or fossa ovarica. It is not uncommon, during attempts to mobilize the ovary to remove the cyst wall, that rupture and release of the contents will occur. In this case, adequate irrigation of the peritoneal cavity is necessary to remove all the cyst contents prior to closure.

In the treatment of ovarian endometriomas, it is essential that the cyst wall lining is excised or destroyed in its entirety to prevent recurrence.

Extrapelvic endometriosis

Sampson[33] originally divided endometriosis into two main groups: direct or internal, adenomyosis, and indirect or external endometriosis. In recent times, most clinicians would think internal endometriosis (adenomyosis) to be of a different aetiological background. Additionally, the indirect external endometriosis is subdivided into pelvic endometriosis and extrapelvic endometriosis. Pelvic endometriosis is defined as endometriotic lesions involving the uterus, ovaries and Fallopian tubes and surrounding peritoneum of the anterior and posterior cul-de-sac and around the pelvic side walls, whilst extrapelvic endometriosis is defined as endometriotic-like lesions elsewhere in the body.

Extrapelvic endometriosis has been found in virtually every organ system and tissue in the human female body. Pelvic and extrapelvic endometriosis are different only in their recurrence rate and anatomical location. Overall, the incidence of extrapelvic disease represents less than 12% of reported cases of endometriosis overall[39]. It would appear that the frequency of occurrence decreases as the distance from the uterus and Fallopian tubes increases[40].

Intestinal tract endometriosis
The intestinal tract represents the highest incidence of extrapelvic disease, with the most frequent area of involvement being the sigmoid colon and rectum, followed by the ileocaecal area and appendix. Less commonly involved are the small bowel and transverse colon.

In the management of endometriosis involving the intestinal tract without obstruction, medical suppressive therapy is most commonly applied. However, with increasing depth of invasion, the serosal surface alone is no longer involved and the muscularis and even the mucosal lining become infiltrated. If this situation occurs, then surgical intervention becomes increasingly likely and more so as the increased fibrotic response within the bowel wall will very often produce subacute or complete obstruction requiring segmental bowel resection.

Presenting complaints of patients with intestinal tract endometriosis are most commonly abdominal pain, followed by distention, bowel function defects and cyclical rectal bleeding. Intestinal obstruction is a frequent finding in more advanced disease and seems to favour the rectosigmoid area.

Urinary tract endometriosis
Endometriotic lesions of the pelvic ureter and bladder are less common than intestinal tract disease but are the next most common sites of extrapelvic endometriosis. Unilateral involvement of the ureter and kidney is the most common form of the disease, but

bilateral involvement can occur. Endometriosis of the urinary tract may occur at any location, with the highest incidence involving the bladder, followed by the lower ureter, the upper ureter and lastly the kidney[41].

Where endometriosis involves the mucosal lining of the urinary tract, it presents, wherever the site of involvement, with haematuria. Common symptoms of vesical endometriosis are dysuria, urgency and frequency, whilst with renal endometriosis the patient commonly presents with haematuria and abdominal pain. Extrinsic ureteral endometriosis eventually induces partial or complete obstruction of the ureter. It is the presence or absence of ureteral obstruction which usually determines surgical management. When obstruction is present, the surgical approach is, wherever possible, segmental resection and reanastomosis or reimplantation of the ureter, although urinary diversion is sometimes necessary.

Involvement of surgical scars

The most common surgical scars involved are those following laparoscopy (umbilicus), abdominal scars following gynaecological procedures or Caesarean section and at the perineum following episiotomy at childbirth. Most patients present with a palpable mass, generally causing pain and usually more symptomatic at the time of menstruation. Occasionally, patients can be referred because of haemorrhage, with a cyclical pattern and occurring perimenstrually.

Medical treatment may control the symptoms over a period of time but wide local excision is normally necessary.

Endometriosis of the vagina following hysterectomy is not uncommon, usually with conservation of one or both ovaries and usually in patients with a past history of endometriosis. It can develop in patients given unopposed oestrogen replacement treatment when oophorectomy has already been performed. When it develops with an intact uterus and ovarian function, these lesions are most commonly found in the posterior fornix. In all but a few instances, these lesions on the vaginal surface are continuous with deep infiltrating disease in the cul-de-sac and rectovaginal septum. Whilst the visible lesion in the vagina can be quite small, the full extent of the involvement can only be appreciated by bimanual pelvic assessment under anaesthesia, and it usually requires laparotomy and open resection to achieve an adequate treatment excision.

Pulmonary and thoracic endometriosis

Endometriosis of the lungs and thorax represents an uncommon site of extrapelvic endometriosis. Diagnosis is usually difficult because symptoms of thoracic endometriosis are similar to those of more common pulmonary pathologies, and presenting symptoms and signs usually include chest pain, pneumothorax, haemothorax or haemoptysis, usually concomitant with menstruation.

Management of pulmonary endometriosis appears to favour surgical intervention with thoracotomy for excision of the lesions and/or pleurodesis[39].

Suppressive hormonal therapy can be used as an interim measure and may help after surgery, but with most deep-seated and extrapelvic endometriosis, recurrence following cessation of hormonal suppressive therapy is the likely scenario, making definitive surgery the preferred choice.

Section 2 Endometriosis Illustrated

List of illustrations

Figure 26
Peritoneum with gland lined by endometrial-like epithelium (high power)
Figure 27
Biopsy of the same patient after GnRH analogue treatment (low power)
Figure 28
Biopsy of the same patient after GnRH analogue treatment (high power)
Figure 29
Biopsy from red papule on day 24 (low power)
Figure 30
Biopsy from red papule on day 24 (high power)

Non-pigmented implants
Figure 31
Small, non-haemorrhagic papules
Figure 32
Less pigmented lesions in association with other features
Figure 33
Biopsy from yellow-brown lesion (low power)
Figure 34
Biopsy from yellow-brown lesion (high power)
Figure 35
Biopsy from white lesion (low power)
Figure 36
Biopsy from white lesion (high power)

Scarified implants
Figure 37
White opacified lesions associated with abnormal vasculature
Figure 38
White scarification with active red lesions
Figure 39
White scarred area, indicating deep endometriosis (distant view)
Figure 40
White scarred area, indicating deep endometriosis (close-up view)
Figure 41
Thickened, white scarified lesion

Figure 42
White scarification in cul-de-sac
Figure 43
White scarred lesions with surrounding increased vasculature
Figure 44
Endometrial lesions overlying a scarified area
Figure 45
Extensive scarification and deep, infiltrating endometriosis

Peritoneal pockets
Figure 46
Peritoneal pouch in cul-de-sac
Figure 47
Peritoneal pouch in cul-de-sac
Figure 48
Peritoneal pocket above left uterosacral ligament
Figure 49
Pseudo-pocket
Figure 50
Peritoneal pouch with obvious endometriosis in base
Figure 51
Peritoneal pouches with associated endometriosis

Adhesions
Figure 52
Increased peritoneal fluid in minimal/mild endometriosis
Figure 53
Filmy adhesions
Figure 54
More extensive adhesions in advanced endometriosis
Figure 55
Extensive adhesions
Figure 56
Complete obliteration of cul-de-sac after previous surgery
Figure 57
Vascularity and haemorrhagic lesions before and after GnRH analogue treatment

Cutaneous endometriosis
Figure 125
Endometriosis in episiotomy scar
Figure 126
Endometriotic deposit in Caesarean section scar
Figure 127
Endometriosis involving the umbilicus
Figure 128
Excision of umbilical endometriotic lesion
Figure 129
Biopsy of endometriosis in skin of abdominal wall
(low power)
Figure 130
Biopsy of endometriotic deposit in skin (high power)

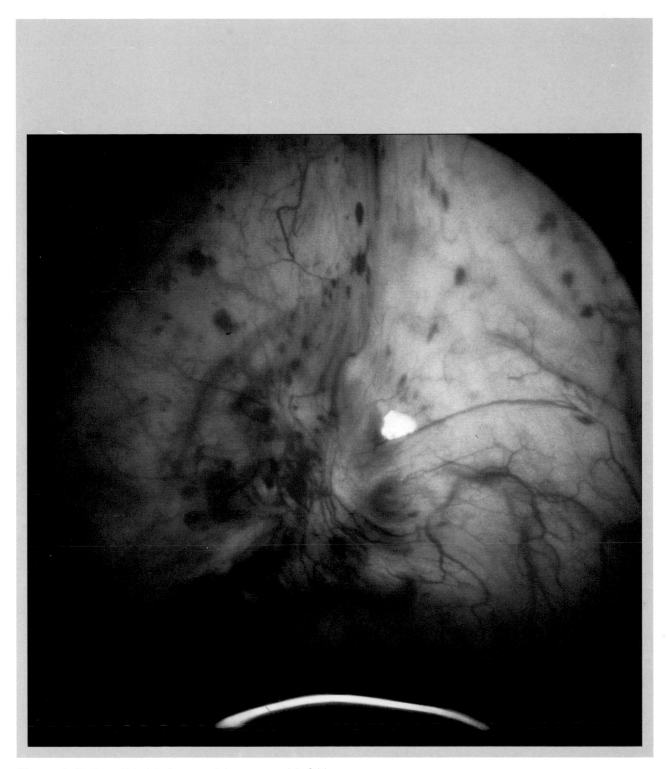

Figure 1 Puckered black lesions overlying uterovesicle fold. These lesions are the classical 'powder burn' diagnostic markers of endometriosis but may represent a less active form of the disease

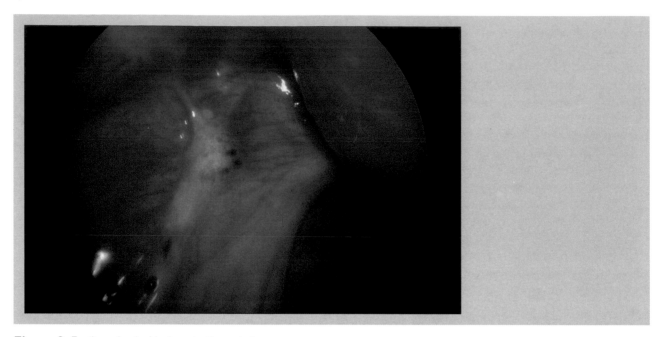

Figure 2 Further classical lesions in the cul-de-sac

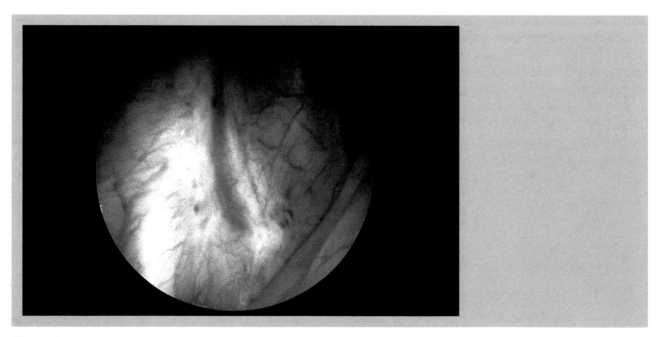

Figure 3 Classical 'powder burn' lesions as seen after 6 months' treatment with Danol

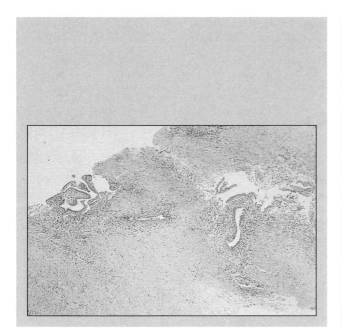

Figure 4 A low-power view of biopsy from lesion overlying uterovesicle pouch, showing fibrous tissue with endometriosis. The glands are inactive and no haemosiderin disposition is seen (biopsy taken on day 21 of cycle)

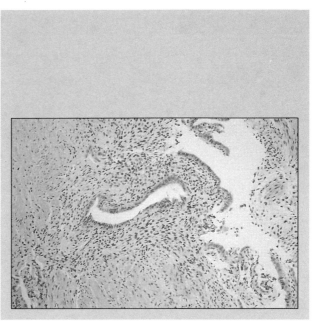

Figure 5 A high-power view of same biopsy as in Figure 4

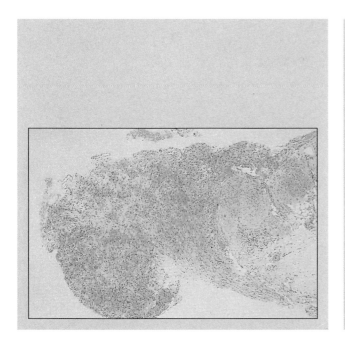

Figure 6 A low-power view of biopsy from black lesions on uterosacral ligament on day 9 of cycle. Section shows fibro-adipose tissue with endometrial-like stroma, recent and old haemorrhage and fibrosis, but no gland formation. This could possibly be a resolving lesion

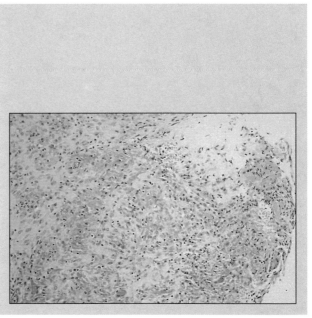

Figure 7 A high-power view of the same biopsy as in Figure 6

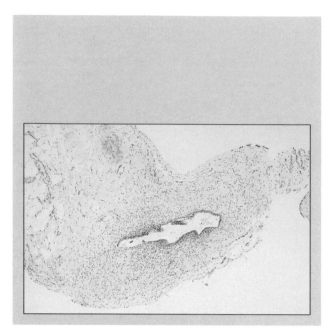

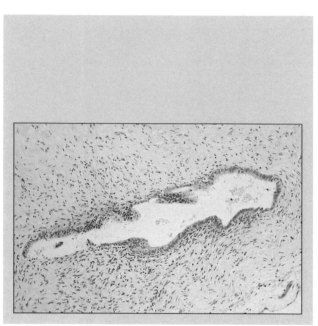

Figure 8 A low-power view of biopsy from left uterosacral ligament, showing pigmented lesion on day 24 of cycle. Fibrous connective tissue with mesothelial covering contains small foci of endometriosis with haemorrhage and chronic inflammation (out of phase with endometrium)

Figure 9 A high-power view of the same biopsy as in Figure 8

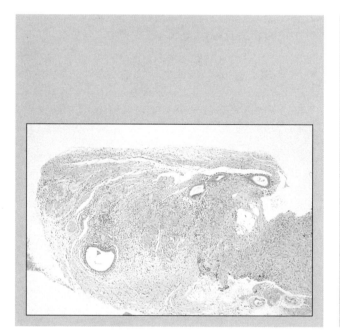

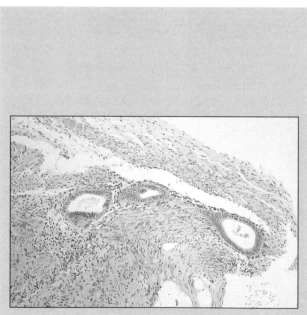

Figure 10 A low-power view of the same patient as in Figures 8 and 9 rebiopsied after 6 months' GnRH analogue treatment. Fibrous tissue contains inactive glands surrounded by a small amount of endometrial stroma. One gland contains haemosiderin-laden macrophages

Figure 11 A high-power view of the same biopsy as in Figure 10

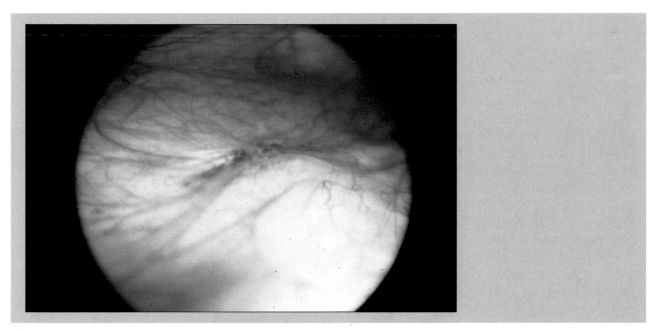

Figure 12 Increased vascularity and haemorrhagic lesions at the peritoneal site of a previous laparoscopy incision in a patient with other features of recurrent pelvic endometriosis. (Photo courtesy of Mr C. Sutton)

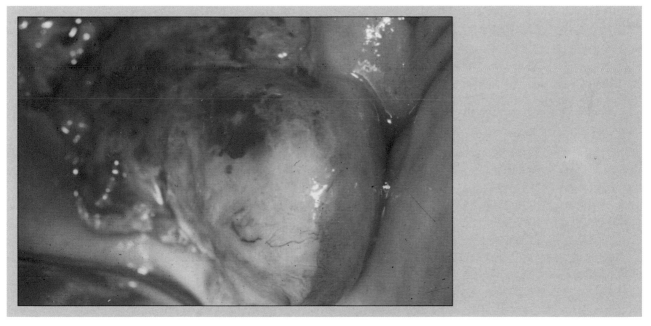

Figure 13 Extensive haemorrhagic lesions, evidence of active, symptomatic disease

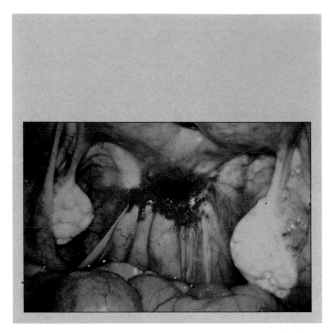

Figure 14 Extensive haemorrhage, associated with deep infiltrating endometriosis involving the descending colon

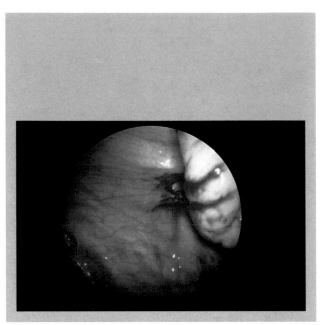

Figure 15 Haemorrhagic lesions and early adhesion formation on posterior lateral border of ovary

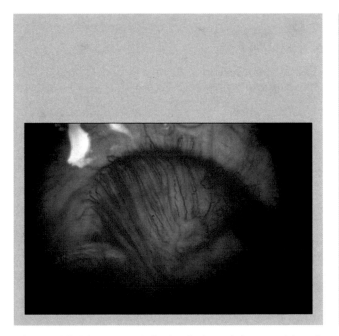

Figure 16 Hypervascularization in the cul-de-sac, with early pseudopouch formation. This is an indication for biopsy to establish diagnosis of endometriosis

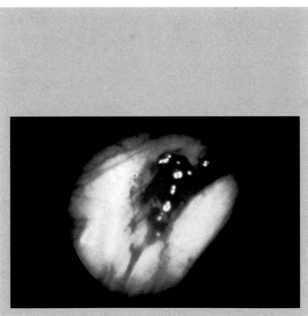

Figure 17 Haemorrhagic bleb on pelvic peritoneal surface indicating likely presence of endometriosis

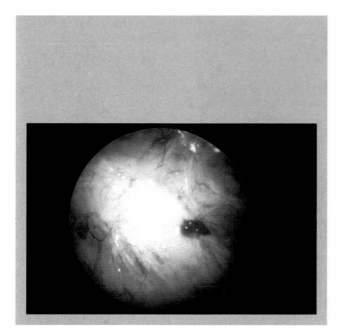

Figure 18 Isolated red lesions, associated with some areas of scarification in patient with recurrent endometriosis

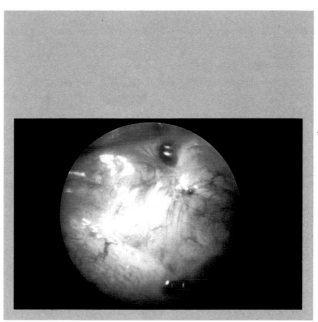

Figure 19 Another example of isolated red lesions

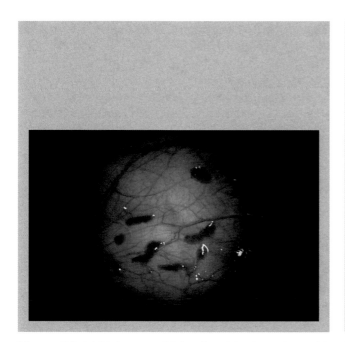

Figure 20 Multiple, superficial red vesicles in patient with biopsy-proven endometriosis

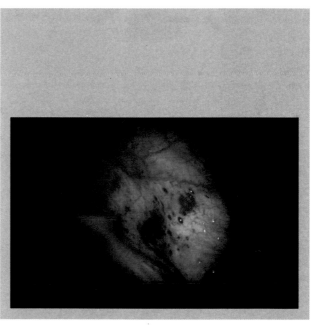

Figure 21 Another example of multiple, superficial red vesicles

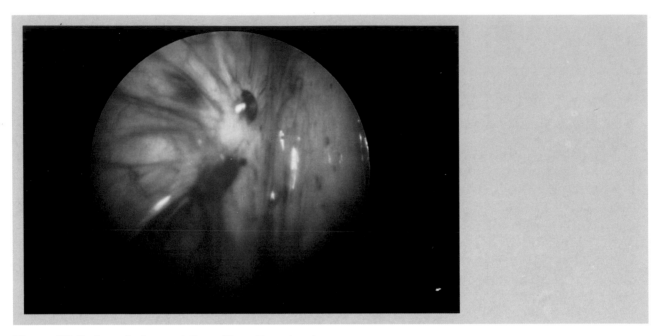

Figure 22 Red papules in association with peritoneal puckering and scarring

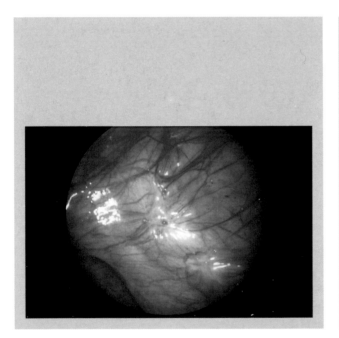

Figure 23 Modification of red lesions, with reduced redness and vascularity following 6 months' treatment with GnRH analogues

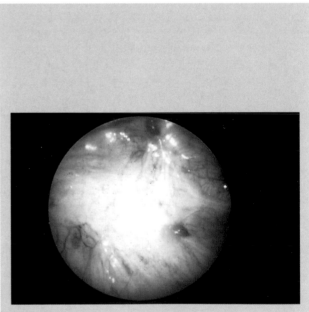

Figure 24 A second example of modification of red lesions

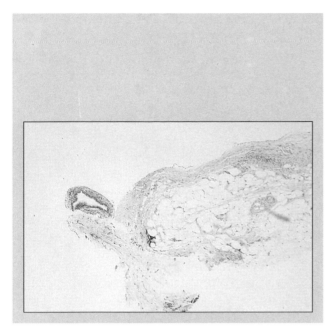

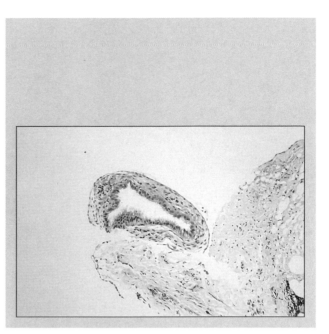

Figure 25 Low-power section of peritoneum with gland lined with endometrial-like epithelium and surrounded by stroma and haemorrhage. Secretory activity is not seen (biopsy on day 15 of cycle)

Figure 26 High-power section of same biopsy as in Figure 25

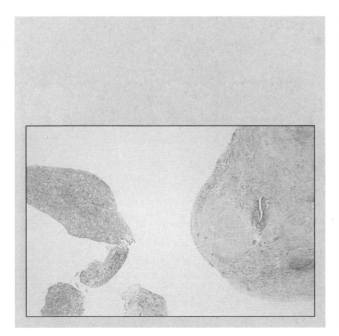

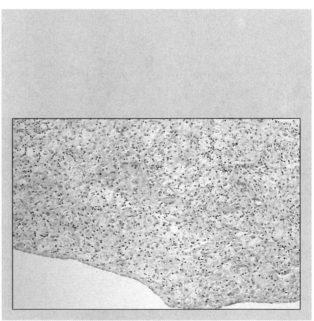

Figure 27 Low-power section of same patient as in Figures 25 and 26 with biopsy at second-look laparoscopy after 6 months' treatment with GnRH analogues. Section shows fragments of connective tissue with endometrial-like glands and stroma with areas of haemosiderin staining in areas of necrosis and within macrophages

Figure 28 High-power section of same biopsy as in Figure 27

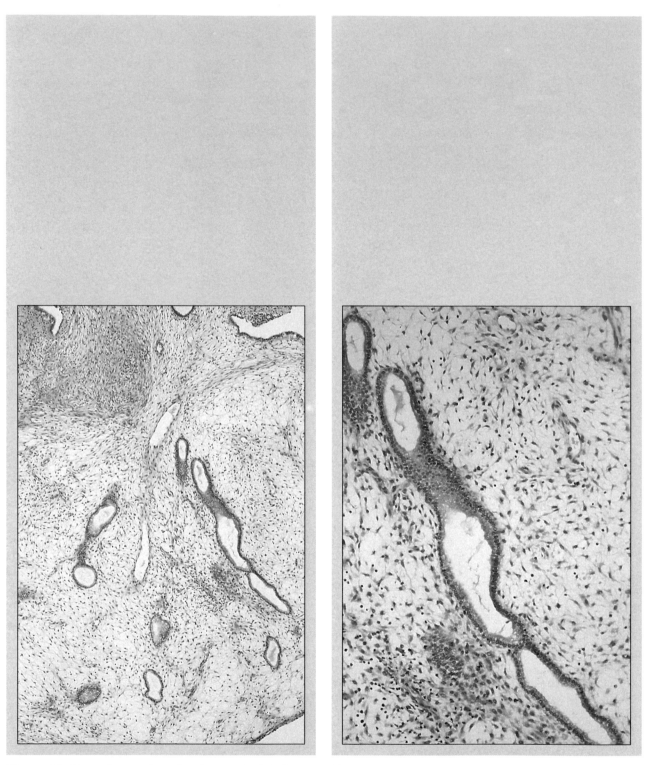

Figure 29 Biopsy from red papule taken on day 24 of cycle. Histology shows oedematous connective tissue including haemosiderin-laden macrophages and glandular structures composed of columnar cells showing secretory activity. Active endometriosis in phase with endometrium (low power)

Figure 30 High-power view of same biopsy as in Figure 29

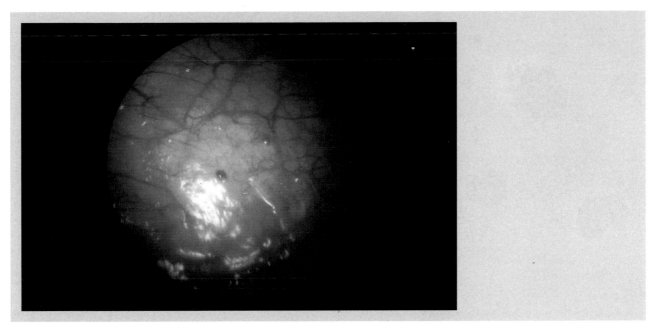

Figure 31 Small, non-haemorrhagic papules may be the first feature discernible laparoscopically in patients with endometriosis

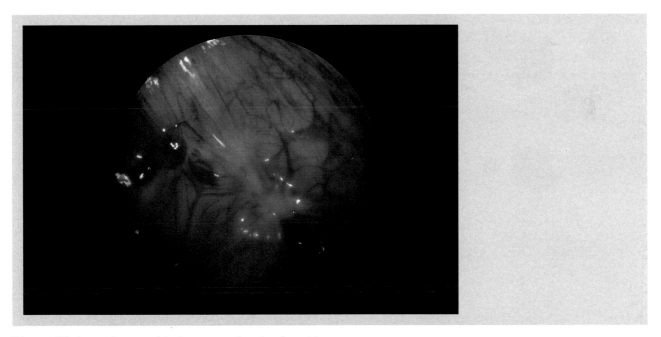

Figure 32 Less pigmented lesions can often be found in association with other features of endometriosis

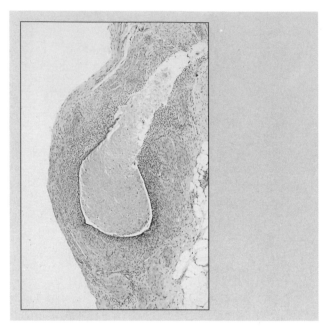

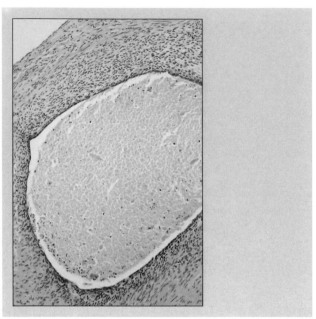

Figure 33 Biopsy from yellow-brown lesion. Low-power section shows fibrous tissue with a small endometriotic gland filled with blood (patient at day 26 of cycle). Features could be described as a 'mini-endometrioma' in the peritoneal lining

Figure 34 A high-power view of the same biopsy as in Figure 33

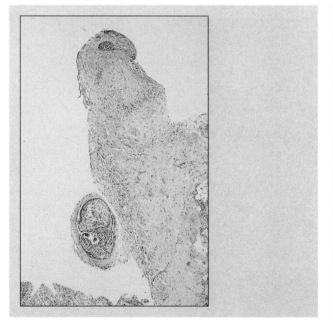

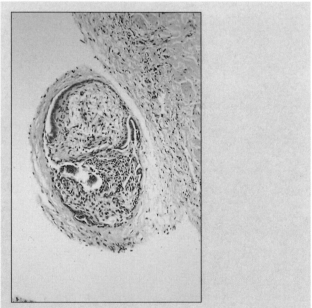

Figure 35 A low-power view of peritoneal biopsy from white lesion on uterosacral ligament on day 22 of cycle. Foci of endometrial glands and stroma are shown embedded in the peritoneum

Figure 36 A high-power view of the same biopsy as in Figure 35

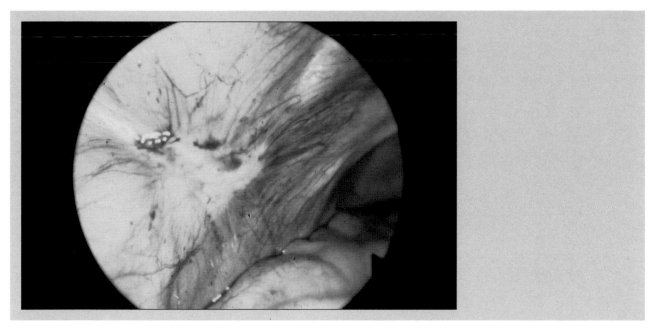

Figure 37 White opacified lesions associated with abnormal vasculature, in this instance in close proximity to the left ureter. (Photo courtesy of Mr C. Sutton)

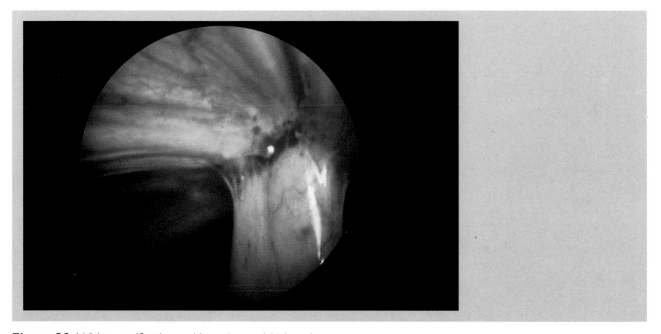

Figure 38 White scarification, with active red lesions involving the right round ligament

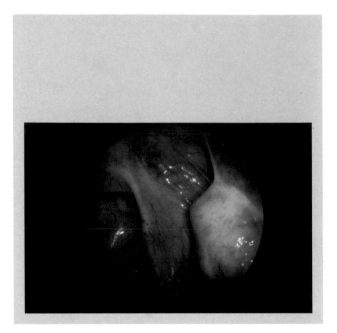

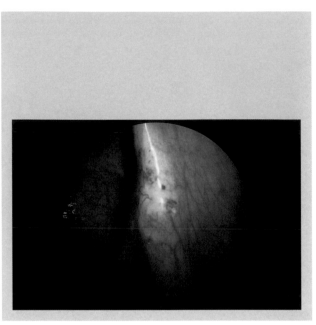

Figure 39 A distant view of white scarred area indicating the presence of deep endometriosis in the right uterosacral ligament

Figure 40 A close-up view of the same white scarred area as in Figure 39

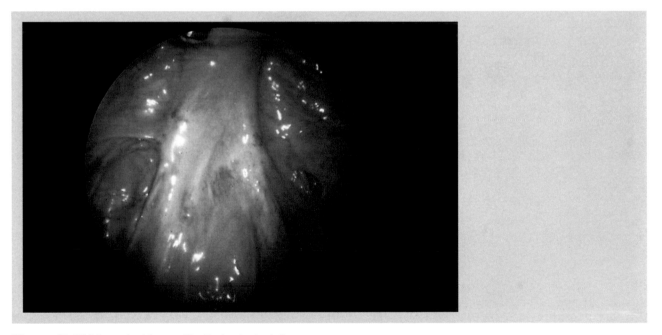

Figure 41 Thickened, white scarified lesion in the left uterosacral ligament

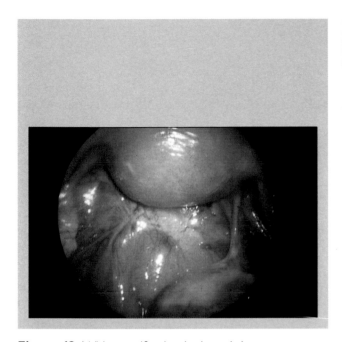

Figure 42 White scarification in the cul-de-sac

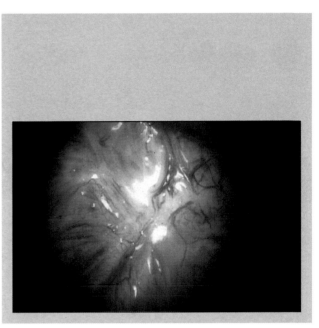

Figure 43 White scarred lesions on the pelvic side wall associated with surrounding increased vasculature

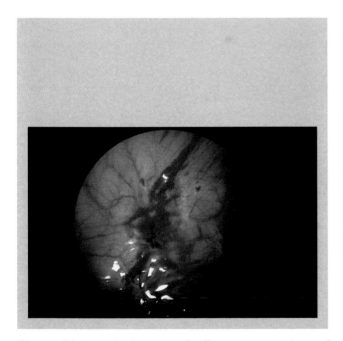

Figure 44 Multiple features of different presentations of endometriotic lesions overlying a scarified area

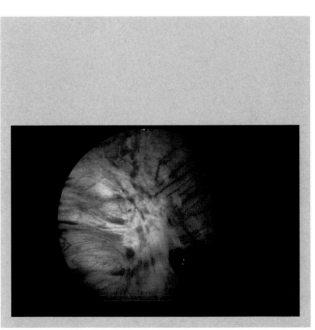

Figure 45 Extensive scarification in association with deep, infiltrating endometriosis

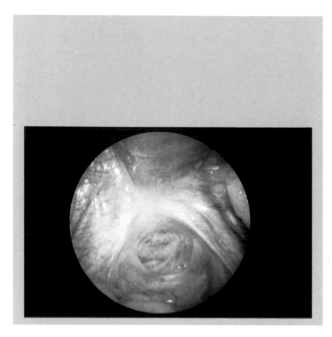

Figure 46 Peritoneal pouch (pocket) in the cul-de-sac

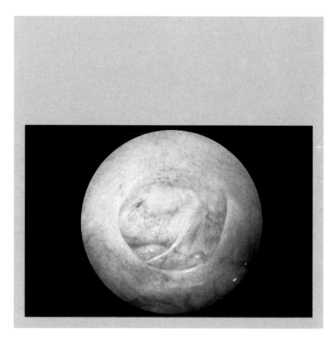

Figure 47 Another example of a peritoneal pouch in the cul-de-sac

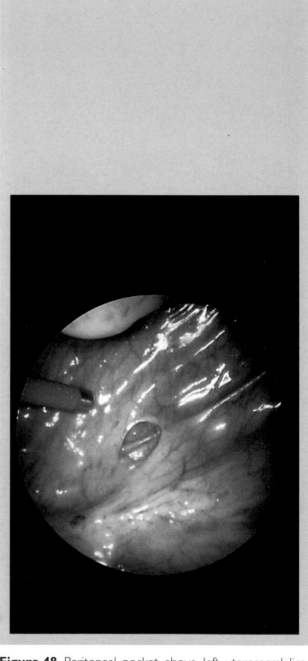

Figure 48 Peritoneal pocket above left uterosacral ligament

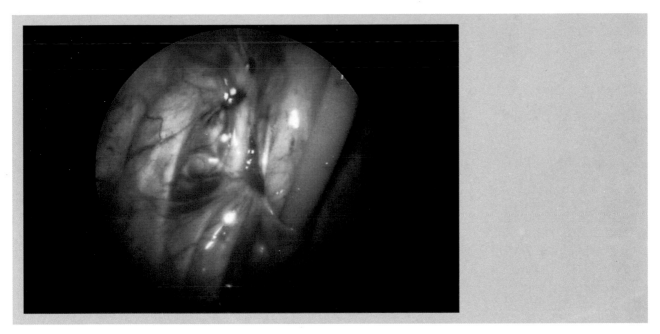

Figure 49 Pseudo-pocket being formed from adhesions around endometriotic deposit

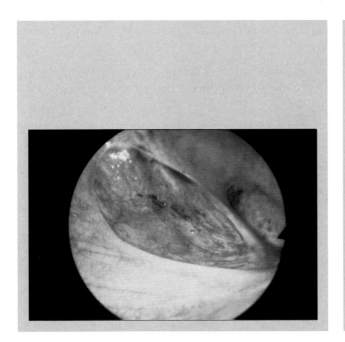

Figure 50 Peritoneal pouch in cul-de-sac with obvious endometriosis in the base. (Photo courtesy of Mr C. Sutton)

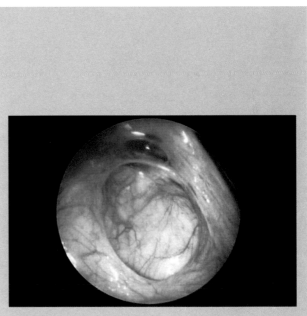

Figure 51 Peritoneal pouches near right uterosacral ligaments with associated endometriosis

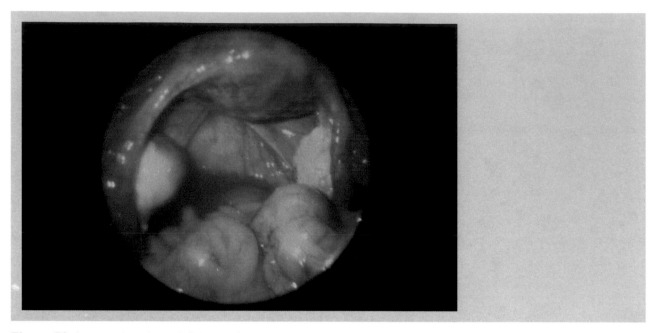

Figure 52 Increased peritoneal fluid is often a finding in patients with minimal and mild endometriosis. It should be aspirated at the onset of the laparoscopy to allow adequate evaluation of the cul-de-sac

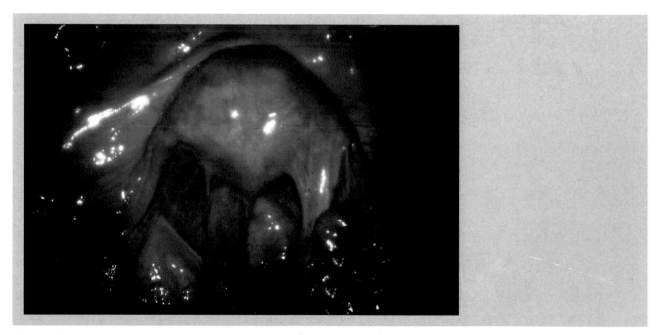

Figure 53 Some filmy adhesions may need to be divided to allow complete evaluation of the cul-de-sac and adnexae

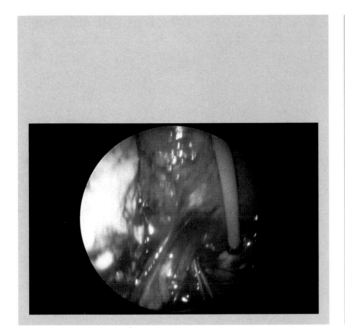

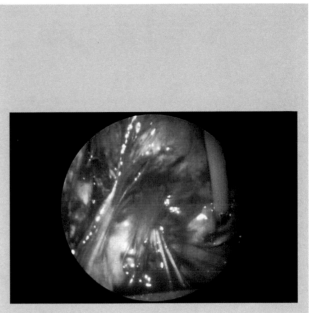

Figure 54 More extensive adhesions are common with advanced endometriosis, especially involving the ovary

Figure 55 Another example of extensive adhesions

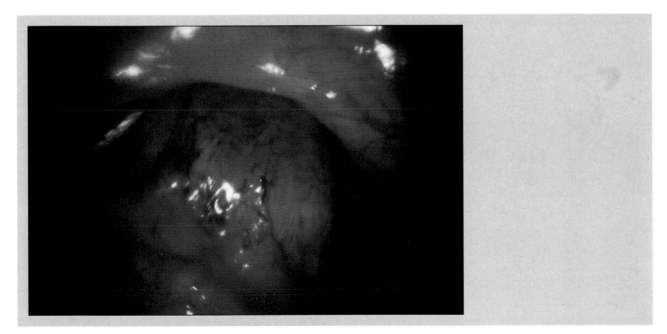

Figure 56 Often following previous surgery, the cul-de-sac can be completely obliterated, making re-evaluation of patients with recurrent symptoms difficult or virtually impossible

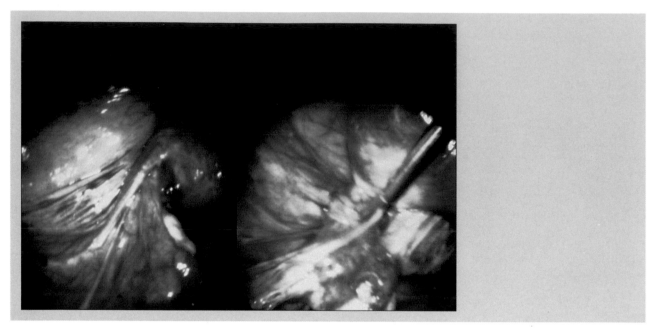

Figure 57 Reduced vascularity of lesions, and disappearance of haemorrhagic lesions pre-therapy (left) and following 6 months' therapy (right) with the GnRH analogue, Synarel. (Photo courtesy of Syntex Pharmaceuticals, UK)

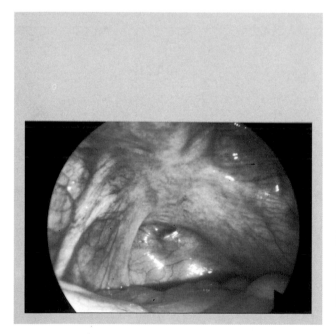

Figure 58 Diffuse endometriosis over thickened uterosacral ligaments

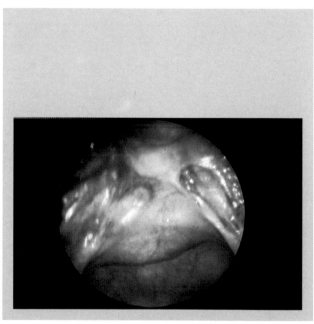

Figure 59 Same area as in Figure 58 as viewed 6 months after KTP laser destruction and laparoscopic laser uterosacral nerve ablation. (Photo courtesy of Mr C. Sutton)

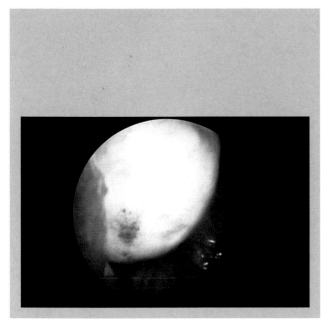

Figure 60 Superficial implant on ovary showing marked reduction in vascularity following 6 months' treatment with norethisterone

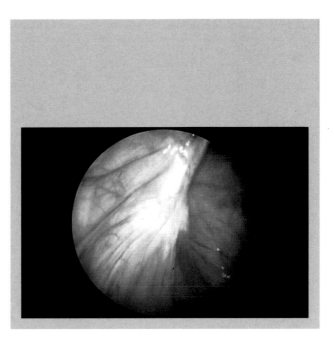

Figure 61 Inactivity and scarring of previously active lesions following 6 months' therapy with GnRH analogue

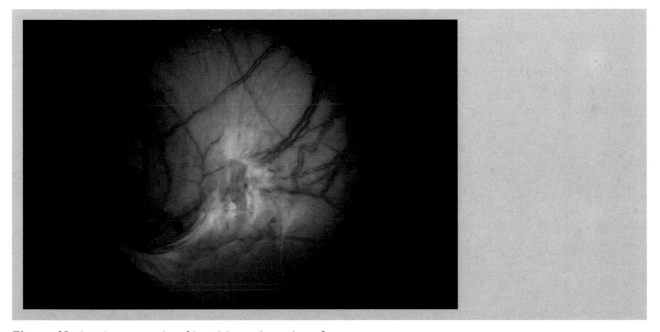

Figure 62 Another example of inactivity and scarring of previously active lesions

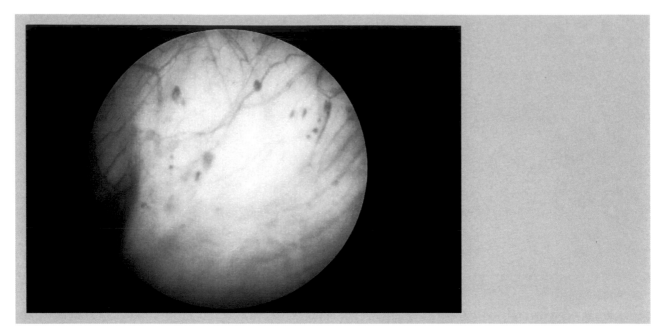

Figure 63 Previous red lesions becoming non-pigmented and associated with scarification following 6 months' treatment with danazol

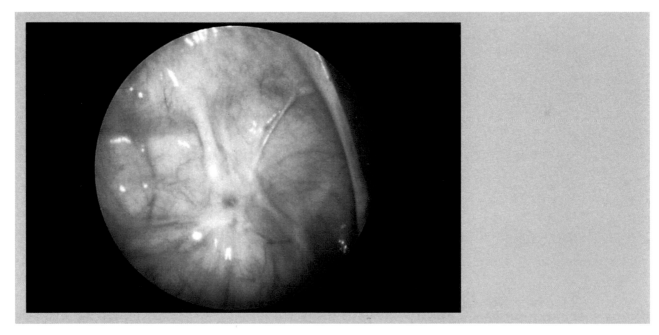

Figure 64 Virtual disappearance of lesion at second-look laparoscopy following 6 months' course with GnRH analogue

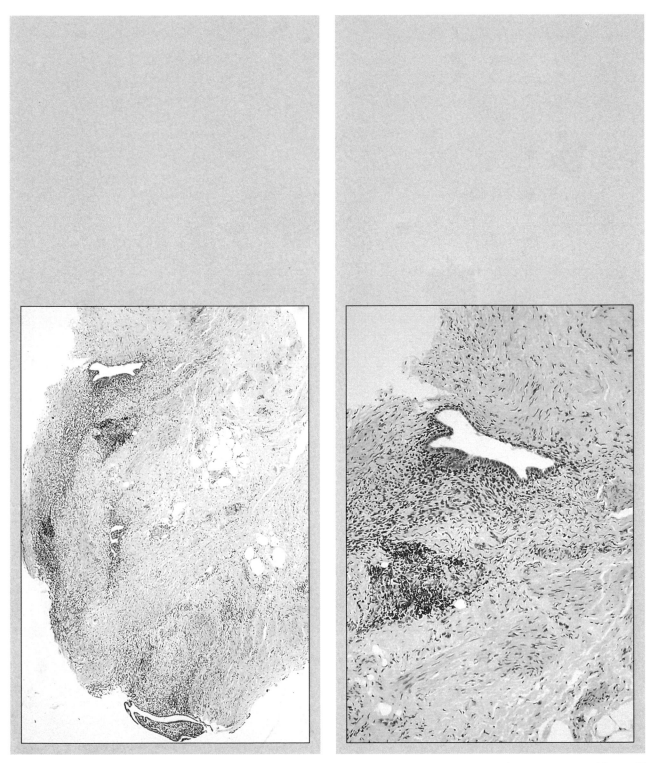

Figure 65 Low-power section of peritoneal biopsy of 'black' lesion after 6 months' treatment with GnRH analogue. Section shows subperitoneal fibroconnective tissue in which are foci of inactive endometriosis

Figure 66 High-power section of same biopsy as in Figure 65

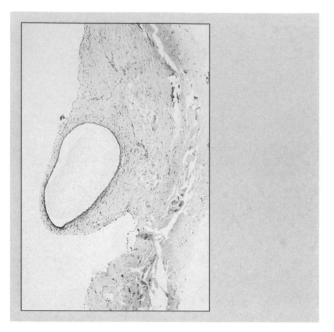

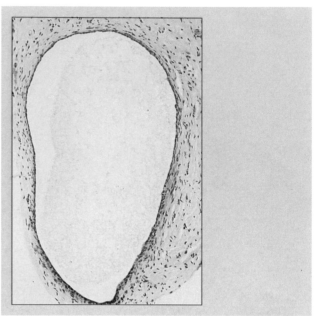

Figure 67 Low-power section of peritoneal biopsy from modified deposit after 6 months' treatment with a GnRH analogue. Section shows fibrous connective tissue with one small (0.8 cm diameter) inactive endometriotic cyst (gland) lined by attenuated epithelium and with only a small degree of surrounding endometrial stroma

Figure 68 A high-power section of the same biopsy as in Figure 67

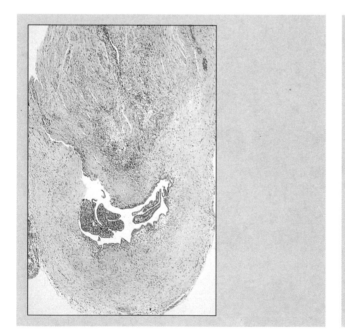

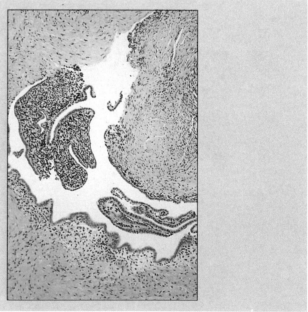

Figure 69 A low-power view of peritoneal biopsy from a non-pigmented modified lesion after 6 months' therapy with a GnRH analogue. Section shows subperitoneal fibroconnective tissue in which there is a focus of endometriosis and a small quantity of haemosiderin

Figure 70 A high-power view of the same biopsy as in Figure 69

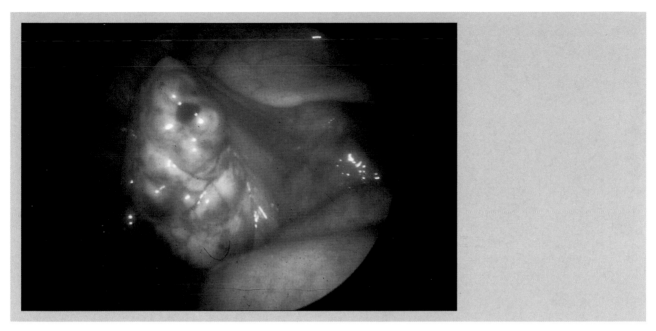

Figure 71 Superficial endometriosis on right ovary

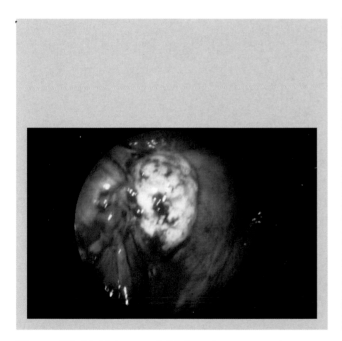

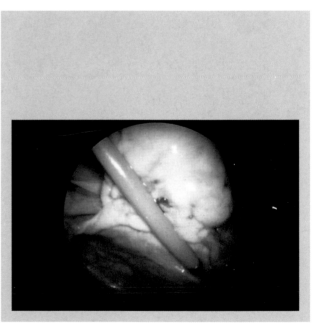

Figure 72 Multiple superficial deposits on posterier aspect of right ovary

Figure 73 Superficial deposits on posterier aspect of right ovary

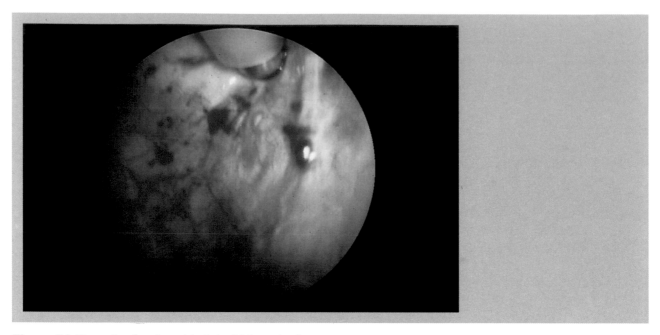

Figure 74 Deposits of endometriosis in right ovarian fossa

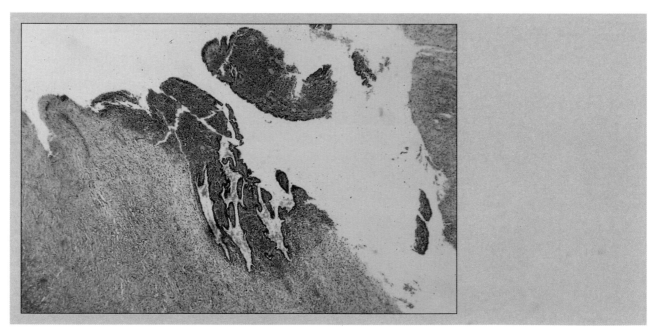

Figure 75 Superficial ovarian endometriosis with a marked haemorrhagic response (H & E × 35)

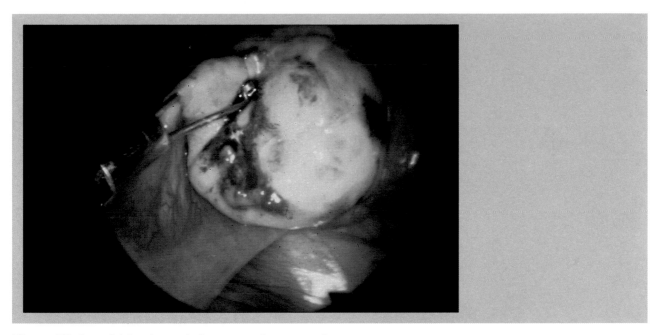

Figure 76 Superficial endometriosis on posterior aspect of ovary before treatment. (Photo courtesy of Mr C. Sutton)

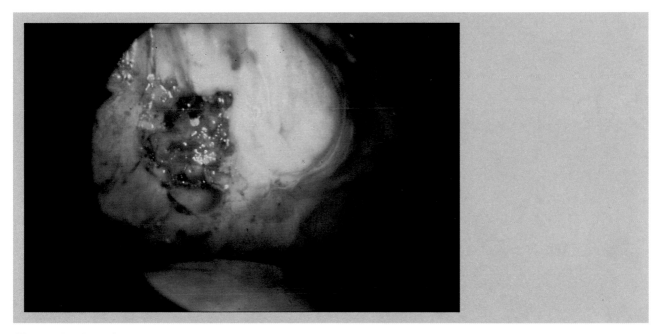

Figure 77 Superficial endometriosis of ovary following vaporization with KTP laser. (Photo courtesy of Mr C. Sutton)

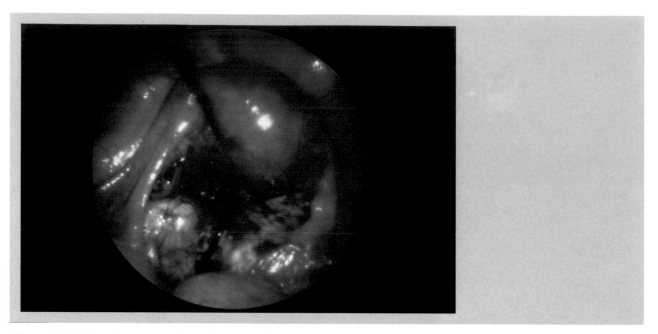

Figure 78 Bilateral ovarian endometriomas, adherent to each other, and posterior uterine wall – 'kissing ovaries'

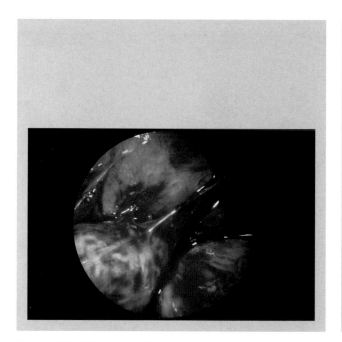

Figure 79 Bilateral ovarian endometriomas, with extensive adhesions and haemorrhage

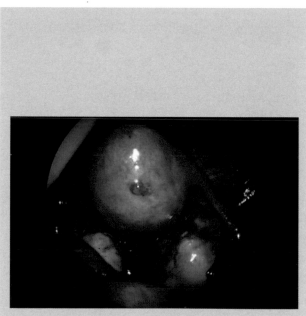

Figure 80 Endometrioma on right ovary

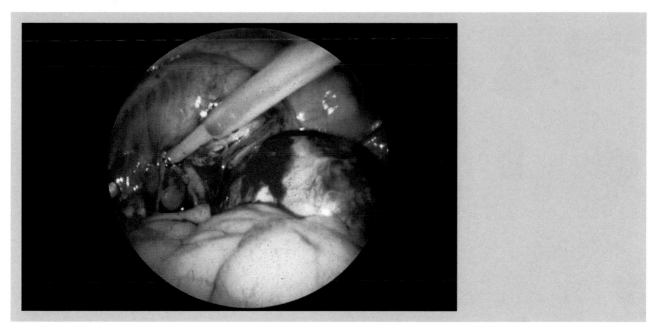

Figure 81 Endometrioma on left ovary, with adhesions to descending colon

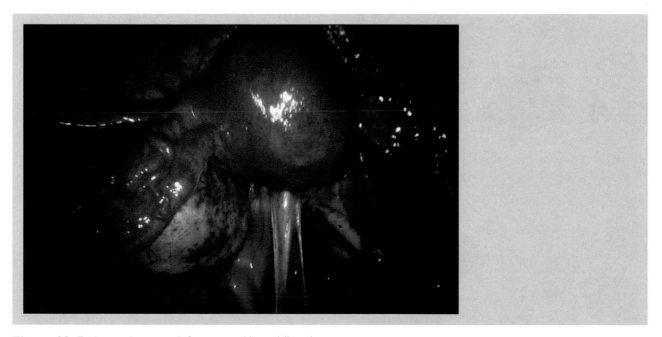

Figure 82 Endometrioma on left ovary, with mobile tube and ovary partially fixed to the posterior leaf of broad ligament and adhesions in the pouch of Douglas

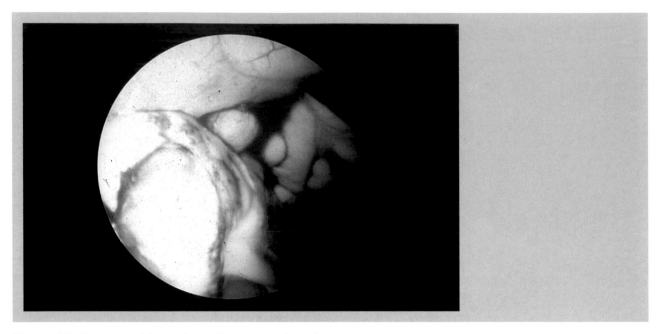

Figure 83 Ovary containing endometrioma approximately 3 cm diameter. Note the presence of increased amounts of haemorrhagic peritoneal fluid, but no other overt features of endometriosis. (Photo courtesy of Professor J. Donnez)

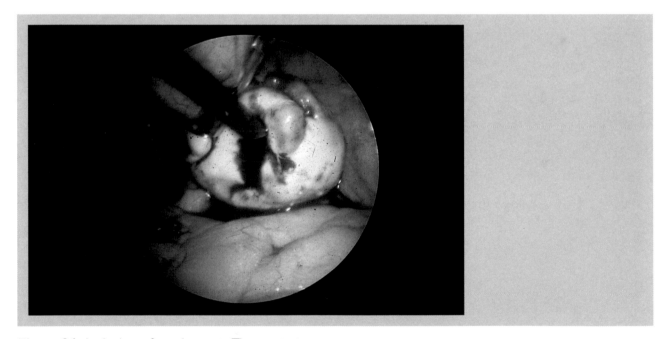

Figure 84 Aspiration of ovarian cyst. The contents are typical of endometrioma. Aspiration is necessary for diagnosis, and as preparation for laparoscopic laser destruction. (Photo courtesy of Professor J. Donnez)

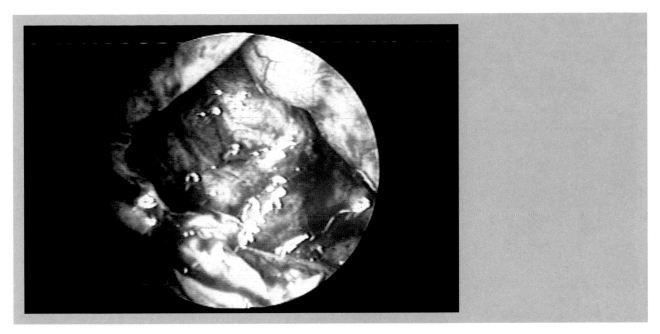

Figure 85 The ovarian endometrioma wall is opened, the contents are aspirated and the cavity washed with normal saline. Note the extreme activity within areas of the cyst wall with local haemorrhage and increased vascularity. (Photo courtesy of Professor J. Donnez)

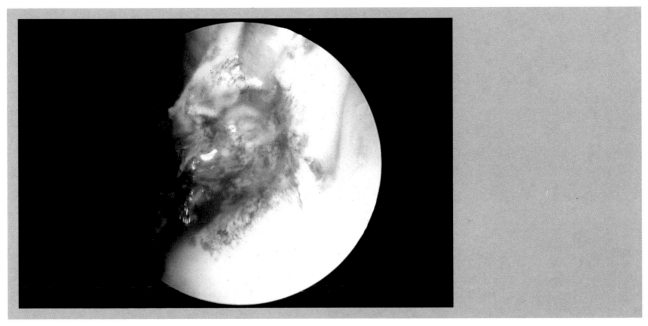

Figure 86 Commencement of CO_2 laser destruction of the internal lining of the endometrioma. (Photo courtesy of Professor J. Donnez)

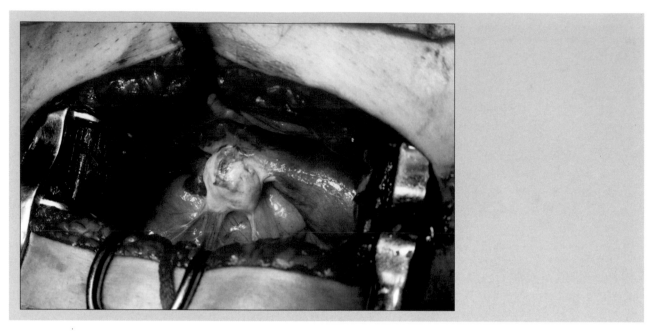

Figure 87 Left endometrioma, pretreated for 4 months with GnRH analogue, with associated adhesions

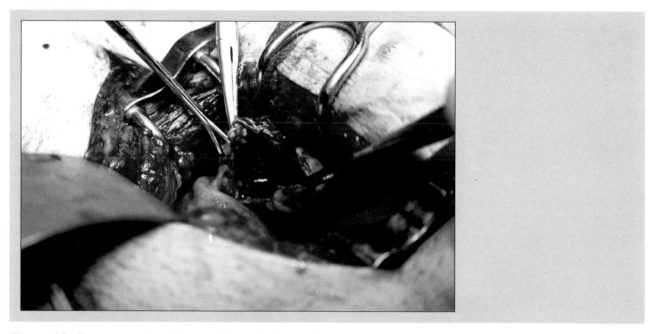

Figure 88 Ovary opened to allow excision of endometriotic cyst lining

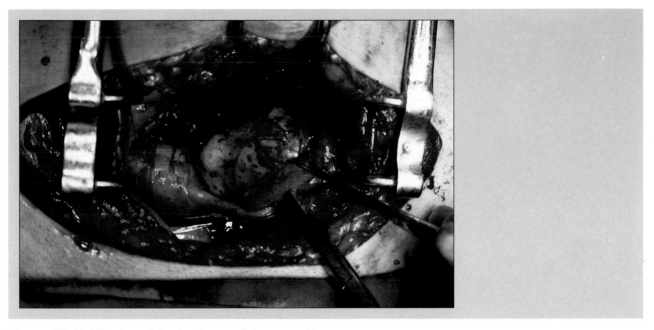

Figure 89 Mobilization of fixed, adherent left ovary with endometrioma

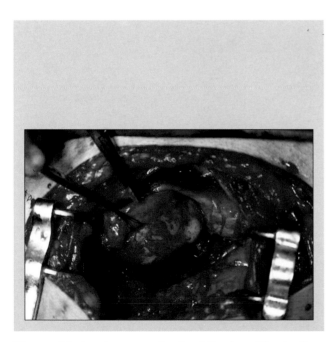

Figure 90 Another example of mobilization of fixed, adherent left ovary with endometrioma

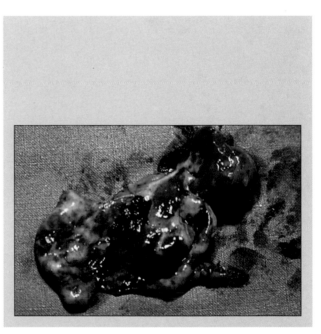

Figure 91 Excised cyst wall of endometrioma

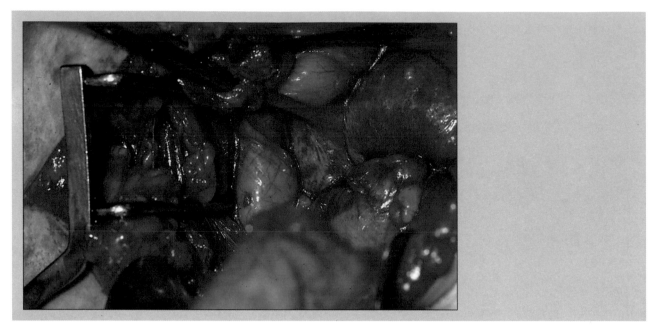

Figure 92 'Frozen' pelvis: extensive adhesions with fixed mass posterior to uterus

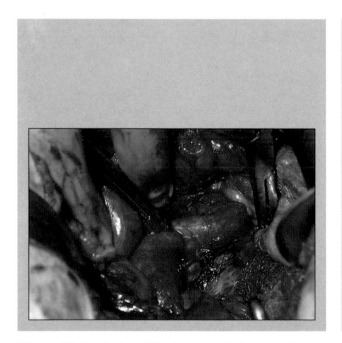

Figure 93 Gradual mobilization revealed enlarged ovary suggestive of endometrioma

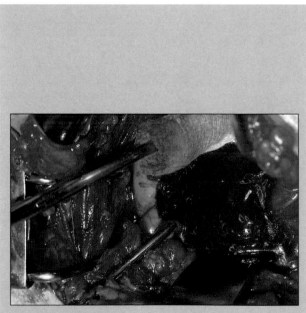

Figure 94 During further mobilization, the cyst ruptured, containing haemorrhagic material. Histology confirmed endometriosis but pelvic damage was extensive and future fertility prospects were viewed as slim

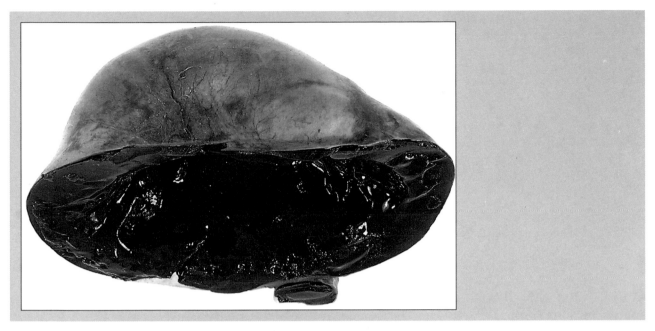

Figure 95 Large endometriotic chocolate cyst of ovary

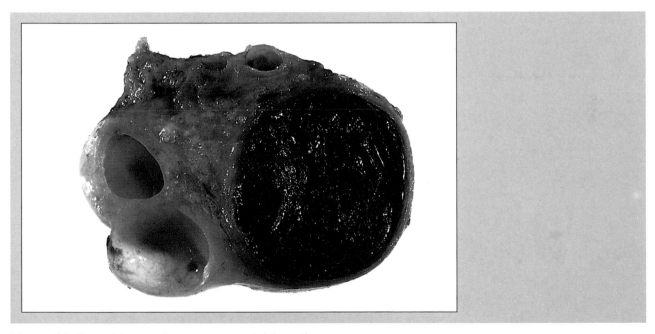

Figure 96 Chocolate cyst in an ovary containing other smaller fibrous-lined cyst cavities

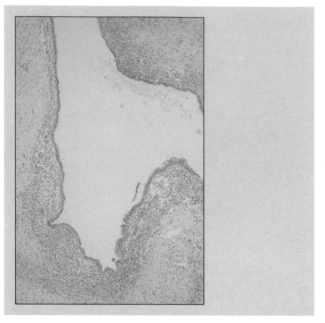

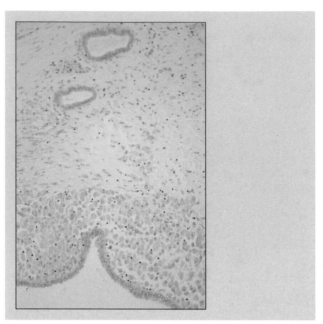

Figure 97 Section from a left ovary containing an endometrioma 3.5 cm in diameter. Section shows endometrial stroma containing endometrial glands, some of which are cystically dilated, and haemosiderin-laden macrophages. Patient had undergone 6 months' pretreatment with a GnRH analogue prior to surgery (low-power × 65)

Figure 98 A high-power view (× 130) of the same left ovary as in Figure 97

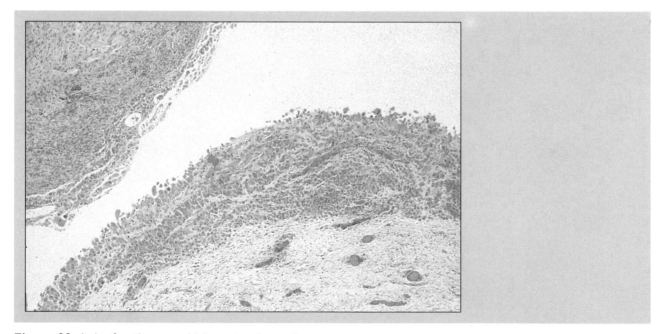

Figure 99 As is often the case with long-standing endometriomas, histology may reveal fibrosis and haemorrhage, haemosiderin-loaded macrophages but no recognizable endometriotic glandular components in a 'classical' clinical endometrioma (H & E × 130)

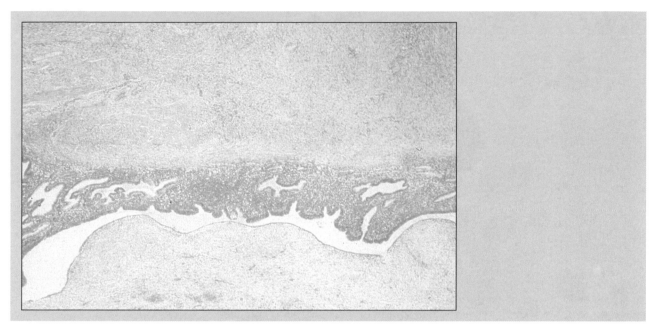

Figure 100 Histology of endometrioma with marked haemorrhage and glandular structures in the cyst wall lining (H & E × 130)

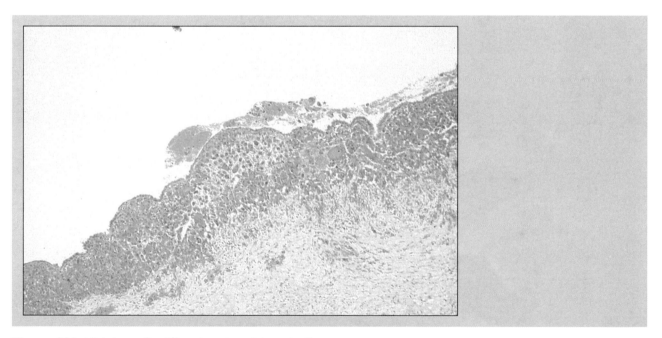

Figure 101 Histology of a different endometrioma to Figure 100, with marked haemorrhage and glandular structures in the cyst wall lining (H & E × 130)

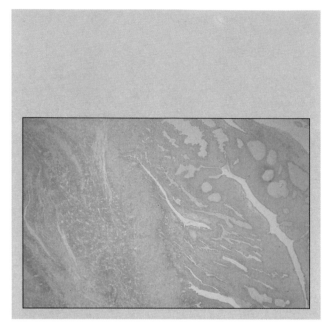

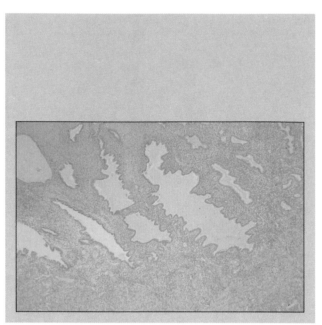

Figure 102 Histology from 4 cm endometriotic cyst in a patient pretreated for 6 months with danazol. There are reduced areas of haemorrhage and the glandular epithelium looks inactive. There are some areas of mucinous metaplasia (low power, × 20)

Figure 103 High-power view of same histology as in Figure 102 (× 80)

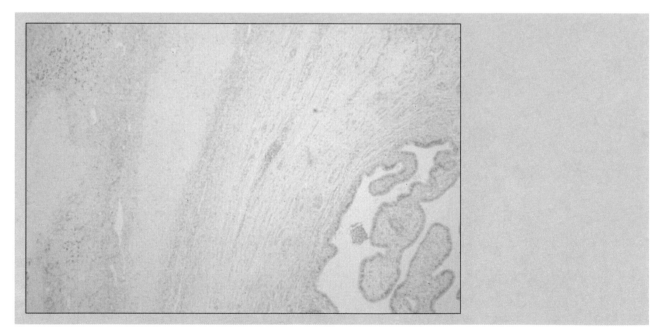

Figure 104 Endometrioma (left) from an ovary which also contained a serous cystadenoma (right)

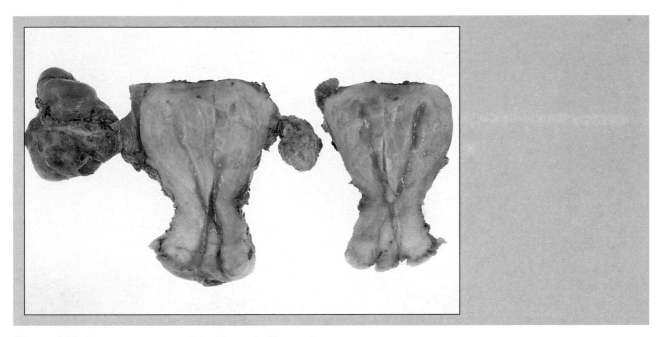

Figure 105 Bicornuate uterus and double cervix. The ovaries contained multiple cysts of endometriotic origin, with endometriosis within the tubal wall in addition

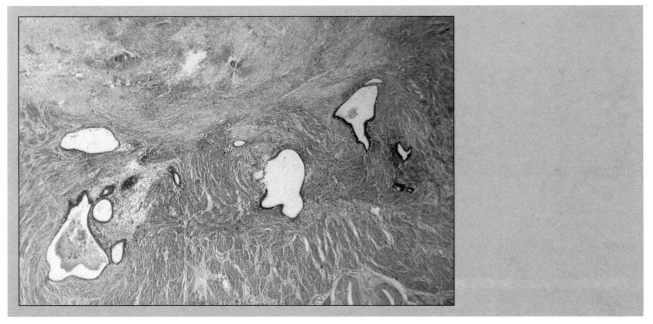

Figure 106 Endometriosis deep within the posterior wall of the uterus (H & E × 35)

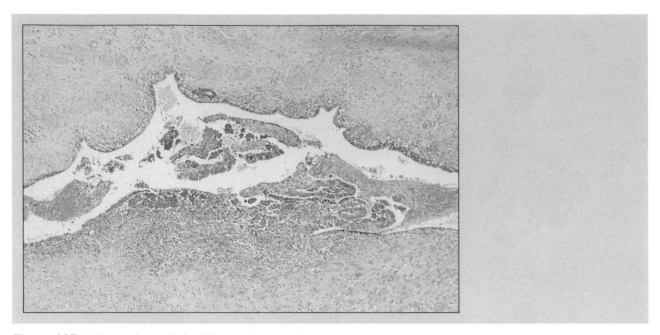

Figure 107 Active endometriosis with recent haemorrhage within the wall of the Fallopian tube (H & E × 130)

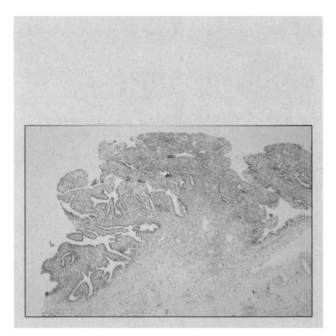

Figure 108 Inactive endometriosis deep to tubal mucosal lining in a patient with ovarian endometriosis operated on after 6 months' treatment with danazol (H & E × 85)

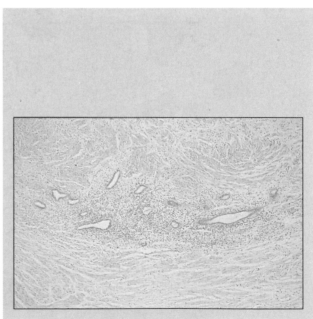

Figure 109 Inactive endometriosis within the Fallopian tube (H & E × 20)

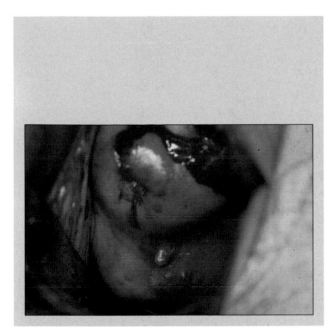

Figure 110 Endometriosis involving the posterior vaginal fornix. This deep endometriosis was continuous with lesions in the pouch of Douglas. (Photo courtesy of Dr D. Bromham)

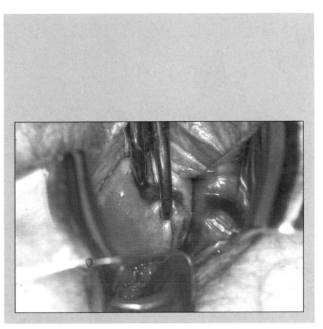

Figure 111 Endometriotic deposits in the posterior vaginal fornix presenting with dyspareunia and postcoital bleeding in a patient with known pelvic endometriosis. The lesions were less obvious since viewed after 4 months' treatment with a GnRH analogue

Figure 112 Excised vaginal vault endometriotic lesion from patient in Figure 111

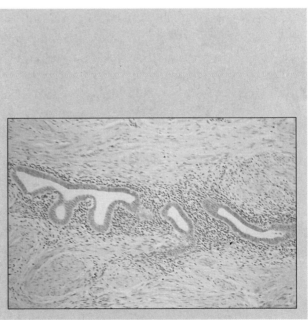

Figure 113 Histology from vaginal vault lesions, with endometriotic foci showing poor activity, but patient had received GnRH analogues for 4 months preoperatively

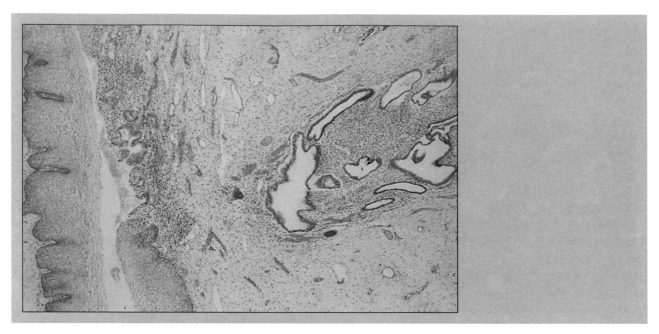

Figure 114 Endometriosis in the cervix found in a patient undergoing loop excision for severe dyskaryotic smear and CIN I on biopsy (low power H & E). An incidental finding at histology

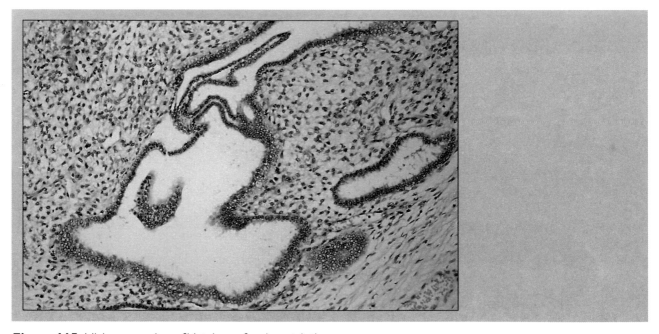

Figure 115 High-power view of histology of endometriotic deposit within cervix showing tubal metaplasia

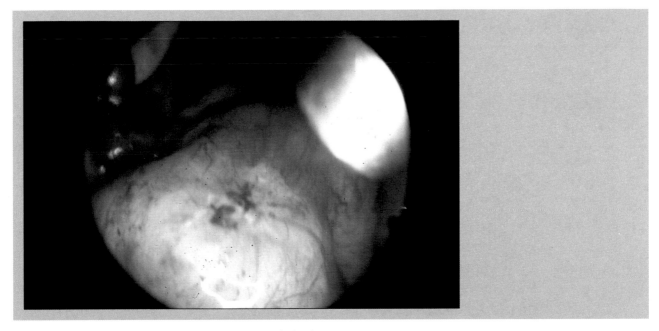

Figure 116 Superficial, vascular active endometriotic deposit on serosal surface of sigmoid colon. One lesion has been vaporized with CO_2 ultrapulse laser. (Photo courtesy of Mr C. Sutton)

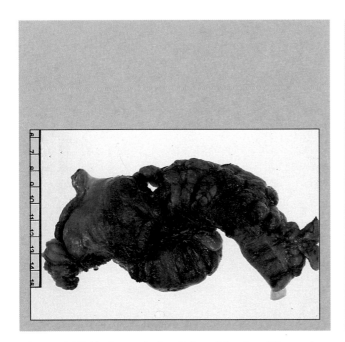

Figure 117 Endometriosis of sigmoid colon. The patient (known to have endometriosis) presented with cyclical rectal bleeding (perimenstrually), increasing dyschaezia and tenesmus, and was admitted with obstruction of large bowel

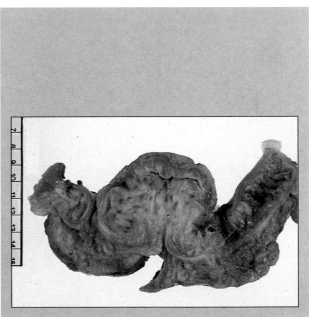

Figure 118 Stricture within colon, increased fibrosis and polypoidal projection of the colon into the mesentary wall with areas of haemorrhage within the wall

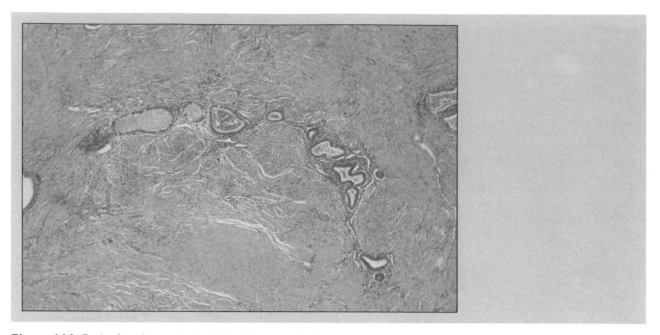

Figure 119 Foci of endometriosis within the muscularis propria of sigmoid colon

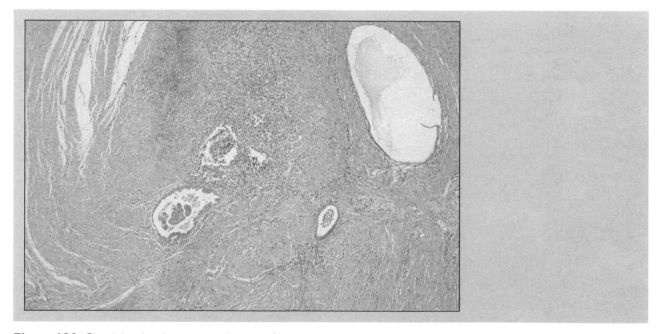

Figure 120 Glandular development and areas of haemorrhage within wall of sigmoid colon

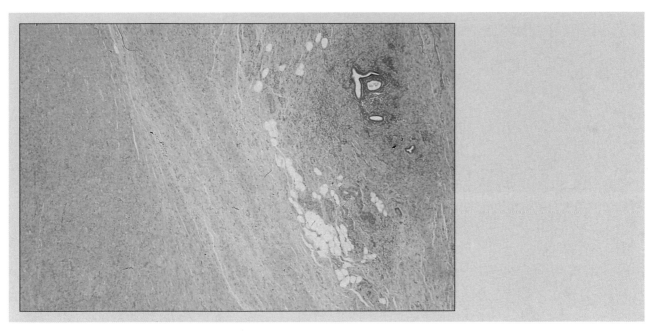

Figure 121 Endometriosis within wall of the appendix, found in a patient undergoing surgery for endometriosis. Low-power view (H & E × 30) with appendix adherent to right ovarian endometrioma

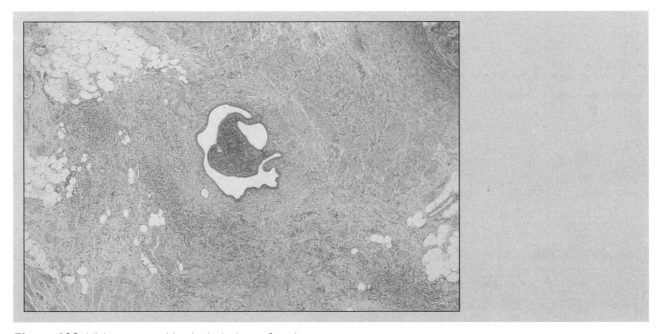

Figure 122 Higher-power histological view of endometriosis involving appendix (H & E × 130)

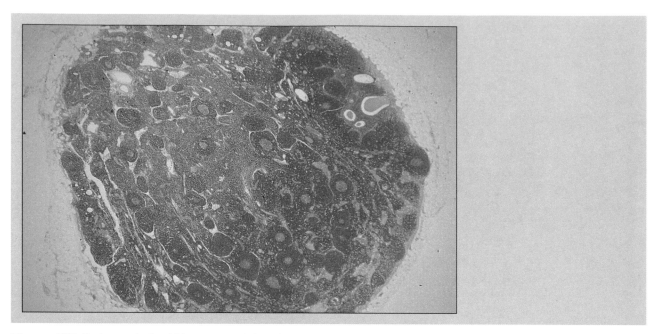

Figure 123 Endometriosis within mesenteric lymph nodes from patient who underwent resection of colon for involvement with endometriosis

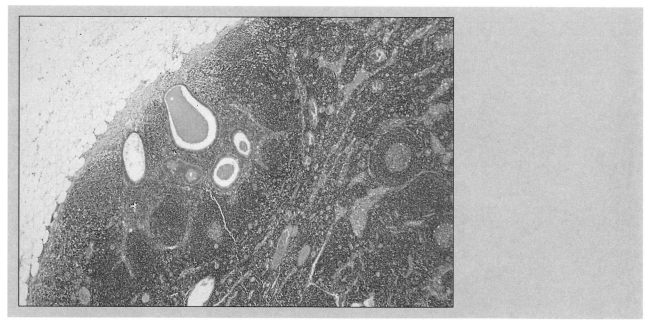

Figure 124 Another example of endometriosis within mesenteric lymph nodes

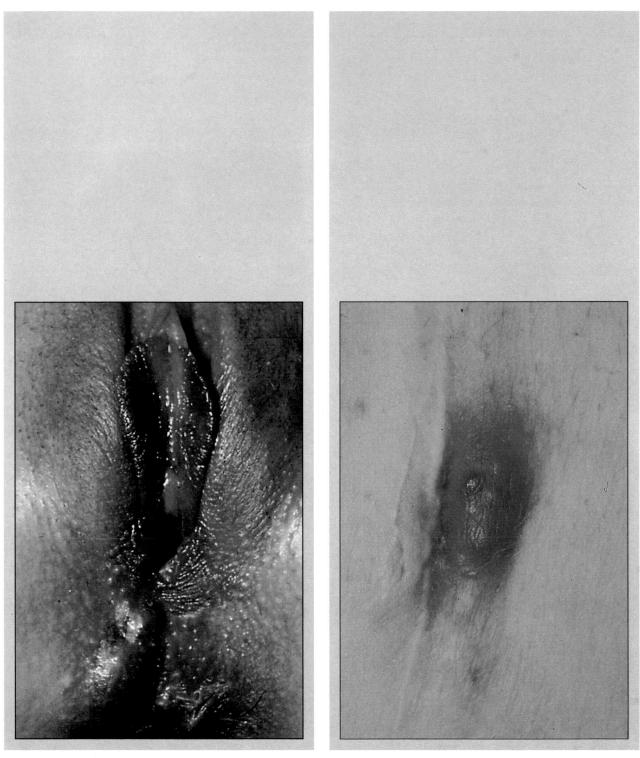

Figure 125 Endometriosis in episiotomy scar. The patient presented with cyclical, tender swelling in the perineum. (Photo courtesy of Mr D. Bromham)

Figure 126 Superficial endometriotic deposit in Caesarean section scar. The patient presented with a cyclical, painful nodule in the scar. (Photo courtesy of Mr D. Bromham and Professor J. Scott)

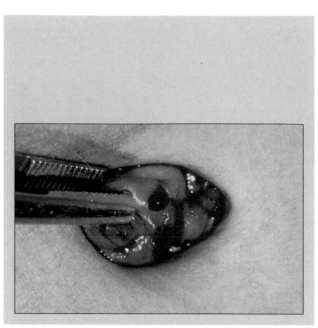

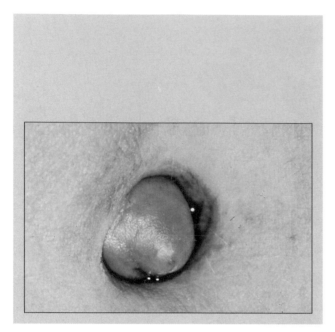

Figure 127 Endometriosis involving the umbilicus in a patient with extensive pelvic recurrent endometriosis. The patient presented with cyclical pain and bleeding from the umbilicus. (Photo courtesy of Mr D. Bromham)

Figure 128 Commencement of excision of umbilical endometriotic lesion. (Photo courtesy of Mr D. Bromham)

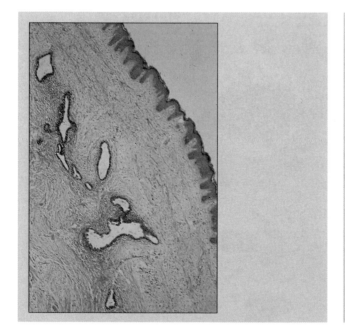

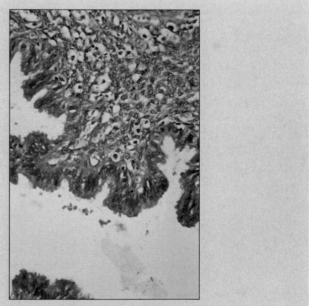

Figure 129 Histology of biopsy from endometriosis in anterior abdominal wall showing glandular elements beneath the skin (H & E × 90)

Figure 130 High-power picture of biopsy from endometriotic deposit in skin, demonstrating glandular structure and macrophages with lipid and haemosiderin accumulation (H & E × 210)

Section 3   Bibliography

1 Jeffcoate, T. N. (1975). *Principles of Gynaecology*, 4th edn., p. 350. (London: Butterworth)

2 Tyson, J. E. A. (1974). Surgical consideration in gynaecologic endocrine disorders. *Surg. Clin. N. Am.*, **54**, 425

3 Strathy, J. H., Molgaard, G. A., Coulam, C. B. and Molton, L. J. (1982). Endometriosis and infertility: a laparoscopic study of endometriosis among fertile and infertile women. *Fertil. Steril.*, **38**, 667

4 Simpson, J. L., Elias, S., Malinak, L. R. and Buttram, V. C. (1980). Heritable aspects of endometriosis. *Am. J. Obstet. Gynecol.*, **137**, 327

5 Kistner, R. W. (1977). Endometriosis. In Sciarra, J. (ed.) *Gynecology and Obstetrics*, Vol. 1. (Hagerstown, New York, London: Harper & Row)

6 DeSanto, D. A. and McBirnie, J. E. (1949). Endometriosis – a clinical and pathological study of 219 cases. *Calif. Med.*, **71**, 274

7 Houston, D. E. (1984). Evidence for the risk of pelvic endometriosis by age, race and socioeconomic status. *Epidemiol. Rev.*, **6**, 167

8 Sampson, J. A. (1927). Peritoneal endometriosis due to menstrual dissemination of the endometrial tissue into the peritoneal cavity. *Am. J. Obstet. Gynecol.*, **14**, 422

9 Schrifin, B. S., Erez, S. and Moore, J. G. (1973). Teenage endometriosis. *Am. J. Obstet. Gynecol.*, **116**, 973

10 Halme, J., Hammond, M. G. and Hulka, J. F. (1984). Retrograde menstruation in healthy women and in patients with endometriosis. *Obstet. Gynecol.*, **64**, 141

11 Dmowski, W. P., Steele, R. W. and Baker, G. F. (1981). Deficient cellular immunity in endometriosis. *Am. J. Obstet. Gynecol.*, **141**, 377

12 Meyer, R. (1919). Veber den Stand der Frage der Adenomyositis, Adenomyome im allegemeinen und insbesondere ueber Adenomyositis seroepithelialis und Adenomyometritis sarcomatosa. *Zentralbl. Gynaekol.*, **36**, 745

13 Levander, G. (1941). Bone formation by induction. An experimental study. *Arch. Klin. Chir.*, **202**, 497

14 Kistner, R. W. (1975). Management of endometriosis in the infertile patient. *Fertil. Steril.*, **26**, 1151

15 Thomas, E. (1991). Endometriosis and infertility. In Thomas, E. and Rock, J. (eds.). *Modern Approaches*

to Endometriosis, p. 113. (Dordrecht, Boston, London: Kluwer Academic)

16 Buttram, V. C. (1979). Conservative surgery for endometriosis in the infertile female: a study of 206 patients with implications for both medical and surgical therapy. *Fertil. Steril.*, **31**, 117

17 Bayer, S. R. and Seibel, M. M. (1986). Endometriosis: clinical symptoms and infertility. In Rolland, R., Chandha Dev, R. and Willemsen, W. (eds.) *Gonadotrophin Down-Regulation in Gynaecological Practice*, p. 103. (New York: Alan R. Liss)

18 Greenblatt, R. B., Dmowski, W. P., Mahesh, V. B. and Scholer, H. F. L. (1971). Clinical studies with an antigonadotrophin – danazol. *Fertil. Steril.*, **22**, 102

19 Schweppe, K. W. (1984). *Morphologie und Klinik der Endometriose*. (Stuttgart, New York: Schattauer)

20 Barbieri, R. L., Bast, R. C., Niloff, J. M., Kistner, R. W. and Knapp, R. C. (1985). Evaluation of a serological test for the diagnosis of endometriosis using a monoclonal antibody OC-125. Presented at the *Annual Meeting of the Society of Gynaecological Investigation*, 33p

21 American Fertility Society (1985). Revised Fertility Society Classification of endometriosis. *Fertil. Steril.*, **43**, 351

22 Acien, P., Shaw, R. W., Irvine, L., Burford, G. and Gardner, R. L. (1989). Ca 125 levels in endometriosis patients before, during and after treatment with danazol or LHRH agonists. *Eur. J. Obstet. Gynaecol. Reprod. Med.*, **32**, 241

23 Acosta, A. A., Buttram, V. C., Besch, P. K., Malinak, L. R., Franklin, R. R. and Vanderheyden, J. D. (1973). A proposed classification of endometriosis. *Obstet. Gynecol.*, **42**, 21

24 Kistner, R. W., Siegler, A. M. and Behrman, S. J. (1977). Suggested classification for endometriosis: relationship to fertility. *Fertil. Steril.*, **28**, 1008

25 American Fertility Society (1979). Classification of endometriosis. *Fertil. Steril.*, **32**, 633

26 Doberl, A., Bergquist, A., Jeppson, S., Koskimies, A. I., Ronnberg, L., Segerbrand, E. *et al.* (1984). Repression of endometriosis following shorter treatment with, or lower dose of danazol. *Acta Obstet. Gynecol. Scand. Suppl.*, **123**, 51

27 Jansen, R. P. and Russell, P. (1986). Nonpigmented endometriosis: clinical laparoscopic and pathological definition. *Am. J. Obstet. Gynecol.*, **155**, 1154

28 Martin, D. C., Hubert, G. D., Vander Zwagg, R. and El-Zeky, F. A. (1989). Laparoscopic appearances of peritoneal endometriosis. *Fertil. Steril.*, **51**, 63

29 Redwine, D. B. (1987). Age related evolution in color appearance of endometriosis. *Fertil. Steril.*, **47**, 1062

30 Brosens, I. A. (1991). The endometriotic implant. In Thomas, E. and Rock, J. (eds.) *Modern Approaches to Endometriosis*, p. 21. (Dordrecht, Boston, London: Kluwer Academic)

31 Sampson, J. A. (1921). Perforating hemorrhagic (chocolate) cysts of the ovary. *Arch. Surg.*, **3**, 245

32 Sampson, J. A. (1924). Benign and malignant endometrial implants in the peritoneal cavity and their relationship to certain ovarian tumours. *Surg. Gynecol. Obstet.*, **38**, 287

33 Sampson, J. A. (1940). The development of the implantation theory for the origin of peritoneal endometriosis. *Am. J. Obstet. Gynecol.*, **40**, 549

34 Vasquez, G., Cornille, F. and Brosens, I. A. (1984). Peritoneal endometriosis: scanning electron microscopy and histology of minimal pelvic endometriotic lesions. *Fertil. Steril.*, **42**, 696

35 Roddick, J. W., Conkey, G. and Jacobs, E. J. (1960). The hormonal response of endometrium in endometriotic implants and in the relationship to symptomatology. *Am. J. Obstet. Gynecol.*, **79**, 1173

36 Schweppe, K. W., Wynn, R. M. and Beller, F. K. (1984). Ultrastructural comparison of endometriotic implants and eutopic endometrium. *Am. J. Obstet. Gynecol.*, **148**, 1024

37 Bergquist, A. (1989). Receptor mechanisms in endometriotic and endometrial tissue. In Shaw, R. W. (ed.) *Advances in Reproductive Endocrinology*, Vol. 1, *Endometriosis*, p. 53. (Carnforth, UK: Parthenon Publishing)

38 Bergquist, A. (1991). Steroid receptors in endometriosis. In Thomas, E. and Rock, J. (eds.) *Modern Approaches to Endometriosis*, p. 33. (Dordrecht, Boston, London: Kluwer Academic)

39 Rock, J. A. and Markham, S. M. (1987). Extra pelvic endometriosis. In Wilson, E. A. (ed.) *Endometriosis*, p. 185. (New York: Alan R. Liss)

40 Williams, T. J. and Pratt, J. H. (1977). Endometriosis in 1000 consecutive celiotomies: incidence and management. *Am. J. Obstet. Gynecol.*, **129**, 245

41 Kerr, S. W. (1966). Endometriosis involving the urinary tract. *Clin. Obstet. Gynecol.*, **9**, 331

Index